Healthy Living
for a
Sharper Mind

**A Clinicians' Guide to Lowering Your
Risk of Alzheimer's Disease and Improving Your Overall Health**

**Featuring recipes from
Pharmacy In Your Kitchen**

**Hayes Woollen, MD
Cheryl Hoover, RPh**

visit us online at
healthylivingsharpermind.com
and
pharmacyinyourkitchen.com

Published by Hayden House, Charlotte, North Carolina

ISBN: 978-0-9994302-9-3 (hardcover)
ISBN: 978-1-7329958-7-1 (paperback)

This book is intended as a reference guide and should not be interpreted as medical advice. The information presented in this book is written as a source of information only and is designed to help you make informed decisions about your health. It is not intended as a substitute for any treatment plan prescribed by your physician. We strongly recommend you consult a qualified medical professional before beginning any new health program. If you suspect you have a medical problem, we encourage you to talk to your doctor. The authors and publisher disclaim responsibility for any adverse effects arising from the use or application of the information contained in this book.

The stories and patient experiences mentioned herein are based on real people. Names and details of experiences have been changed to protect their identities. Likenesses or similarities to stories of people you may identify with are purely coincidental.

Design by Diana Wade
Cover photo and photos on p. 82 and p. 126 by Rusty Williams Photo
Additional interior photos by Cheryl Hoover

*To our children, whose amazing minds are at the beginning of a life
full of learning and wonder.
And to our spouses, Susan and Hunter,
for their enduring patience, love, and understanding.*

Contents

Introduction

We all worry. About our jobs, our children, our retirement savings, the economy, our political climate, global warming . . . our health!

We worry about old age and wonder if it's coming on too quickly. We worry that our minds may not be as sharp as when we were younger. How many of us have gone into a room and forgotten what we were supposed to be doing, or where we put our car keys, and worried it might be a symptom of Alzheimer's disease?

You may have had a relative who had dementia, may have seen their declining health, and worried something similar might be in your future. You might just have normal age-related issues but fear they could turn into something worse. You might have just turned fifty and realize it's likely you now have more years behind you than ahead of you, yet there is still so much you want to do.

As a primary care physician within a large healthcare system, I became increasingly frustrated with how modern medicine was practiced. It seemed as though I was always behind, checking boxes on our electronic medical record, and running through a schedule that routinely packed in thirty-five-plus patients per day. Think about that. I was expected to see one to two patients every ten to fifteen minutes! I can tell you that it's extremely difficult to play a meaningful role in a patient's health when you see them for—at most—ten minutes at a time.

A typical annual physical covers only a small range of basic measurements, blood pressure, weight, standard blood tests, and then you're out the door. You're handed a prescription for anything new that might have come up, like high blood pressure, diabetes, or high cholesterol. You're told to lose some weight and come back in six to eight weeks.

Most of my patients were exceptionally loyal and understanding, but we all felt there had to be a better way. I began to look at our healthcare system as a whole and realized that we aren't really a *health*care system at all. Our healthcare system was designed to take care of the sick. We are a *sick*care system!

Traditional medicine in the United States is exceptional at treating patients who suffer with acute, life-threatening illnesses and specific age-associated diseases. Researchers have uncovered cures to many forms of cancer that were once incurable. Cardiologists can treat atherosclerotic heart disease with stents and coronary artery bypass grafts. Diabetes can be controlled with effective drugs. And powerful antibiotics and antiviral medications can treat infectious diseases that were once considered deadly. Yet the incidence of these diseases continues to rise at unprecedented rates.

Recent studies by the World Health Organization have shown that even though our healthcare spending runs in the trillions of dollars—greater than that of any other country in the world—we rank at the absolute bottom of the list in terms of overall health and outcomes. Our healthcare costs continue to soar in this country, and yet we are one of the *sickest* places to live. We can do better!

The intent of this book is to share with patients, family, friends, and readers what we, as clinicians, have learned about the long-term effects of nutrition, exercise, stress, and sleep on our brains and our overall health. Although hundreds of books have been written on similar subjects over the years, it is sometimes difficult to sort truth from myth regarding how exercise and food affect our bodies—and our minds.

You may be surprised to learn that research has shown that Alzheimer's disease starts twenty and sometimes thirty years *before* any symptoms are noticed. The great news is that the progression of this disease can be significantly influenced by our lifestyle choices. Dr. Chuck Edwards of Memory and Movement Charlotte sums it up best: "We know now that Alzheimer's disease is a slow process that occurs over decades . . . and it is dependent not only on genes and family history, but on how one lives his life."

Clearly, the health of our brains is directly related to the lifestyle decisions we make every day, and it is without doubt that each of us can make a difference in how we age. By improving your diet, exercising regularly, reducing your stress, getting a good night's sleep, and keeping your brain active, you can dramatically reduce your risk of getting Alzheimer's disease. In addition to protecting your brain with these better lifestyle choices, you reduce your risk of getting other diseases, such as heart disease, diabetes, certain cancers, and strokes. By making some changes in your daily habits and reducing the levels of inflammation in your body, you can not only look and feel better, but you can actually improve your overall health.

Billy's experience with our *Healthy Living for a Sharper Mind* program illustrates its value. Billy is a sixty-year-old male who manages a hedge fund. A numbers genius his whole life, he was having increasing difficulty interpreting data charts and spreadsheets. He was constantly tired at work, often falling asleep at his desk, and he was often forgetful. His wife noticed that their bridge games with friends were becoming frustrating for both of them, as he sometimes forgot which suit was trump! The scariest moment came when Billy was driving back from their mountain house in the middle of the day and fell asleep at the wheel, sending his car careening down the side of a mountain. Fortunately, he survived, suffering only some bruised ribs from the airbags. He was lucky.

When we met Billy in our office, we found him to be moderately overweight. His cognitive evaluation revealed low concentration, significant short-term memory lapses, and poor recall. After a thorough history and a comprehensive physical with our team, which included an in-depth nutritional assessment, sleep studies, labs, and neurologic studies, we immediately put Billy on our program. We developed a nutritional plan and exercise regimen, and treated his previously undiagnosed sleep apnea. On his follow-up visit just six weeks later, Billy stated that he was back to enjoying bridge, he was no longer falling asleep on the job, and his performance at work was back to normal. In just forty days, he had lost over fifteen pounds and said he felt better than he had in years.

Healthy Living for a Sharper Mind provides information based on clinical evidence, cutting-edge research, and years of experience with thousands of patients and families. We will discuss how you can protect your brain from the ravages of Alzheimer's disease. Did you know that scientists are increasingly aware that Alzheimer's has many of the same lifestyle origins as heart disease and diabetes? In fact, some clinicians now link Alzheimer's disease to what is known as "type 3 diabetes" because of the high incidence of insulin resistance and inflammation among Alzheimer's patients.

We'll discuss genetic factors that can increase your risk of heart disease as well as dementia. But we also want you to understand that you have the ability to significantly affect the expression of your genes. As Dr. Graham Simpson states in his book *Well Man*, "We are not prisoners of our genetic destiny. Medicine is now beginning to recognize that the key to successful aging is the control of silent inflammation."[1] And there is nothing more powerful at reducing the amount of inflammation in your body than eating healthy foods and exercising regularly.

Numerous studies around the world have shown that eating a Mediterranean-style diet, getting daily physical activity, and not smoking can improve your overall lifespan by more than fourteen years. We suggest that you can also reduce your chances of getting Alzheimer's disease and enhance your brain function by following the recommendations found in this book.

Your overall health is largely determined by many of the lifestyle choices you make every day. In fact, by the time you reach the age of fifty, lifestyle factors account for more than 70 percent of your health and longevity. In other words, lifestyle trumps genes! We now know that of all the genes that directly affect Alzheimer's disease, 95 percent can be dramatically influenced by diet, exercise, sleep, stress, and brain stimulation. By following the program in this book, you can positively impact the expression of your genes and improve your overall health. We have seen firsthand the impact this program has had on people's lives. We have developed personalized plans for many of our patients and have seen their health and quality of life improve after just a few months. Our comprehensive, multimodal approach to brain health incorporates evidence-based, cutting-edge strategies specifically designed to maximize your overall health and mental function.

Healthy Living for a Sharper Mind will help you discover not only why but *how* to make food choices that will create a healthy body and a revitalized brain. You will learn to eat well and will feel better than you have in years. You'll make healthy choices not because you have to, but because you will want to when you realize how much better you feel. You'll have the flexibility to make smart choices from a wide selection of foods without compromising taste or the enjoyment of eating. Our goal is to add years to your life and, more importantly, life to your years.

We hope to change your perception of how the brain ages and what you can do to help prevent memory loss as you grow older. What you're about to learn can make you feel and look better by guiding you to make better dietary decisions, to exercise more, and to get enthusiastic about your health. As a wise physician and friend told us, "It doesn't matter how much money you have or how many things you accumulate in this life if you're not healthy enough to enjoy them." Good luck in your journey to better health and a sharper mind.

—Hayes Woollen, MD

About This Book

This book is designed to help people approaching middle age lose weight, boost their energy, reduce their levels of inflammation, and most importantly protect their hearts and brains. We will not only explain the warning signs and symptoms of Alzheimer's disease, but reassure you that there are many things you can do to prevent the disease from happening. Whether you will develop Alzheimer's disease *can* be influenced by your genes. But we now know that whether or not you have genes that *can* increase your risk, your odds of getting this disease can be dramatically influenced by your lifestyle choices and your environment.

First you will learn how Alzheimer's progresses; in part I, you will come to understand more about the disease and your risk factors for it. Part II gives you the tools you need to start taking action to lower your chances of getting dementia. Part III breaks down what an anti-inflammatory diet is and why it's important, then offers recipes for different types of food you can eat that will help your body heal itself. A list of additional resources at the back of the book may offer further assistance.

PART I

What Causes Alzheimer's Disease?

CHAPTER ONE

What Is Alzheimer's Disease?

Alzheimer's disease is a shadowy abyss
that disengages a person from the world.
—Joseph Jebelli

*Y*ou might have heard the saying, "Of all the things I've lost, I miss my mind the most." Alzheimer's disease deprives people of their minds. They lose their ability to remember their loved ones, enjoy conversation, read novels, see movies, travel, and even, as the disease progresses, the ability to take care of themselves. The devastation of Alzheimer's disease affects more than 40 million people around the world and is expected to affect more than 115 million people by year 2050. In the Unites States alone, 5.8 million people have been diagnosed with Alzheimer's disease, and by 2050, this number is projected to rise to nearly 16 million.

Alzheimer's is the sixth-leading cause of death in the US. In fact, one in three seniors dies with Alzheimer's disease or other forms of dementia. The disease kills more people than breast cancer and prostate cancer combined. While the incidences of most common chronic diseases—cardiac disease, diabetes, cancer, and stroke—have declined in recent years, deaths due to Alzheimer's have increased by as much as 85 percent in the last decade. In 2020, Alzheimer's disease will cost this nation more than $300 billion, and by 2050, these costs could rise as high as $1.1 trillion.

Alzheimer's disease is the most common form of dementia, which means a decline in mental ability, accounting for 70 percent of all cases of dementia. By definition, Alzheimer's disease is a slow, progressive deterioration and shrinkage of the brain, characterized by a decline in thinking and reasoning skills.

The earliest symptom of Alzheimer's is subtle memory loss, especially difficulty remembering recently learned information. Other memory problems include difficulty finding words, not knowing common facts (such as the name of the current president), and disorientation (such as getting lost in one's own neighborhood). As the disease progresses, patients often have difficulty planning and managing tasks such as paying bills and grocery shopping. They may experience unpredictable mood swings. Families often notice personality changes and a lack of motivation. A person with Alzheimer's might become more withdrawn or more easily frustrated by everyday tasks. People with Alzheimer's are eventually unable to perform activities associated with daily living, such as eating, bathing, and using the bathroom.

By examining brain tissue of Alzheimer's patients who died from their disease, we know that Alzheimer's disease is, in part, caused by years of accumulation in the brain of sticky synapse-destroying plaques made of a protein called beta-amyloid. These killer proteins spread and hollow out areas in the brain, causing widespread destruction in places like the hippocampus, the region in the brain crucial for memory, and disrupt the electrical signals that enable us to produce new memories. As these protein plaques grow, they give rise to tangles, deformed proteins that begin to unravel the structure of the brain itself. The ensuing neurotoxic process causes the brain's immunity system to activate, causing an inflammatory storm within the brain. One by one, neurons in the brain die, disrupting not only a person's memories, but also their mood, their facial recognition, and their sense of self. Over the course of this late-stage disease process, the brain often shrinks to the weight of an orange, losing mass at three to four times the rate of a normally aging brain.

According to the Alzheimer's Association, a person's risk of developing this disease doubles every five years after age sixty-five. That means nearly half of all people over age eighty-five have Alzheimer's disease. It is estimated that every sixty-five seconds someone in the US develops this disease.

We now know that by the time a person is diagnosed with Alzheimer's disease—when that person goes, say, from being a high-powered executive to not recognizing his wife of thirty years—the disease process has been going on in his brain for at least twenty, maybe even thirty years. And unfortunately, this advanced stage of brain deterioration is when most clinical trials occur. By this point in the process, the patient has already suffered years of irreversible brain damage.

For years and sometimes decades before a person dies of this fatal disease, Alzheimer's robs its victims of their very humanity and sends their families into turmoil. In his book *The End of Alzheimer's*, Dr. Dale Bredesen, a leading researcher of dementia, sums it up: "Their memories, their capacity for thought, their ability to live full and independent lives—all gone, in a grim and unrelenting descent into a mental abyss where they no longer know their loved ones, their past, the world, or themselves."[2]

Alzheimer: Not a What but a Who

The first person described as having this illness was Auguste Deter, a fifty-six-year-old woman with (at the time) a rather peculiar and inexplicable mental disorder. Auguste began to forget things. She wandered aimlessly around her apartment, misplaced family possessions, forgot how to cook and clean. Her husband, Karl Deter, eventually took his wife to one of the more highly regarded psychiatric clinics in the world, the Asylum for the Mentally Ill and Epileptic—nicknamed the Castle of the Insane—in Frankfurt, Germany. Here, Auguste first met with Dr. Aloysius "Alois" Alzheimer, in 1901.

Dr. Alzheimer was twenty-four when he began his residency at the Castle of the Insane, where he was eventually promoted to senior physician. During his time there,

Alzheimer studied psychiatry and his life-long passion, neuropathology. He introduced large consultation rooms where doctors could talk and develop a dialogue with the patients, and dedicated special rooms to the microscopic examination of brain tissue. In this setting, Alzheimer spent hours hunched over his microscope and became fascinated by the clinical side of psychiatry.

During this time, Alzheimer connected with Dr. Franz Nissl, a distinguished neurologist from Munich. Nissl had been working on a technique he'd discovered as a medical student years earlier. Using a variety of chemical dyes, Nissl stained thin slices of brain tissue to examine the structures in the brain. The details of individual nerve cells were suddenly visible in bright colors under the microscope. The "Nissl stain" became the gold standard in brain science, used by scientists around the globe to show details of nerve cells never seen before: their size, shape, position, and internal components.

According to his notes, on November 26, 1901, Alzheimer was working late at the asylum. The newly admitted Auguste Deter caught his attention for the way she would appear calm and lucid one minute, combative and confused the next. Over the next few months, Auguste became increasingly disoriented, forgetful, and mentally confused. Dr. Alzheimer was fascinated by her condition and became obsessed with her case, believing that there was something in Deter's brain that might be causing these symptoms. This was a radical concept at the time, as most scientists believed this type of dementia to be a psychiatric issue, addressable through psychoanalysis.

Upon Deter's death on April 8, 1906, Dr. Alzheimer had her medical records and her brain brought to his new lab in Munich. Alzheimer immediately noticed how small Deter's brain had been at the time of her death. There was significant loss of tissue throughout the cerebral cortex, the top layer of the brain, seemingly due to the death of nerve cells. Bordering this area of the brain, Alzheimer observed what looked like scar tissue. And when he peered down his microscope, he noticed the presence of numerous scars: plaques and tangles of an unknown substance, varying in size and shape and surrounding the shriveled brain cells.

He saw this as biological evidence for a brain disorder that had previously been classified as purely psychological. Clinically, Deter's illness seemed like a form of dementia, but the deeply bizarre and unique pattern of pathology suggested this was a distinct disease in its own right.

On November 3, 1906, Alzheimer addressed a hundred fellow psychiatrists at the annual South-West German Psychiatrists' meeting in Tubingen, Germany, to discuss his findings and present his patient, the late Auguste Deter. He confidently presented his paper: *On a Peculiar Disease of the Cerebral Cortex.* By connecting the pathological findings of Auguste Deter's brain to the bewildering clinical state of her behavior, Alzheimer challenged his peers to rethink the way they approached this disease. Instead of being rooted in psychology, he emphasized that dementia may, in fact, be caused by a complex riddle of neurobiology. The attendees at the lecture seemed wholly uninterested in what he had to say, but following the talk, a determined Dr. Alzheimer published a short paper summarizing his lecture.

The disease became known as Alzheimer's disease in 1910, when Dr. Emil Kraepelin so named it in the chapter on "Pre-Senile and Senile Dementia" in the eighth edition of his *Handbook of Psychiatry.* By 1911, Dr. Alzheimer's description of the disease was being used for diagnosis by physicians all over the world.

Alzheimer's and Aging

The rate of Alzheimer's disease goes up with age. According to Alzheimers.net, one in ten Americans older than sixty-five has Alzheimer's, and two-thirds of those patients are women. The risk doubles about every five years after that. After age eighty-five, the risk is of developing Alzheimer's disease is nearly 50 percent. African Americans are more than twice as likely as white Americans to have the disease, while Hispanics are 1.5 times more likely to get the disease than white Americans. And with baby boomers getting older, the number of Alzheimer's patients is expected to rise. By 2050, it's estimated there will be sixteen million people living with Alzheimer's. Unfortunately for all of us, this increased risk comes at the time of life when we want to kick back and enjoy the fruits of our hard labor and our retirement savings.

Alzheimer's Is a Decades-Long Process

Most people generally think of Alzheimer's dementia as a disease of elderly people. The truth is, however, that Alzheimer's is not a disease of old age, but a process that starts in middle age, long before it shows any outward signs of deterioration. The disease is caused by many biological processes that overlap and come together over time, causing the buildup of amyloid and the degradation of healthy neurons in the brain.

In their book *The Alzheimer's Solution*, Drs. Dean and Ayesha Sherzai describe four interconnected processes that are responsible for most of the processes in the brain that lead to Alzheimer's and related dementias.

The first is inflammation. Inflammation is a naturally protective function of the immune system for fighting harmful bacteria and viruses and other organisms that may "invade" the body. Acute inflammation is what you see when you cut your finger and you get redness and swelling as blood flow increases to the injured area and facilitates healing. This type of inflammation is essential. Without it, we couldn't heal. Chronic inflammation, on the other hand, is detrimental, and occurs when the inflammatory response is activated long term, often because of constant irritants like high intakes of foods that can cause inflammation, like sugar. Instead of being protective, chronic inflammation is destructive, damaging tissue instead of healing it. The body actually attacks itself when inflammation goes unchecked.

The second process is oxidation. Oxidation occurs naturally when oxygen reacts with other substances and changes them. When an apple left on the kitchen counter turns brown, that's oxidation. The same thing can happen in our bodies and our brains.

Oxidation results in the formation of oxidative byproducts called free radicals. Free radicals are molecules that are unstable and highly reactive and can cause all sorts of destruction within our bodies. Cancer is an example of free radicals gone awry. Because the brain works harder than any other organ in the body—consuming 25 percent of the body's oxygen—it is especially vulnerable to these oxidative reactions. Though the brain has special cells and molecules that help break down and neutralize free radicals, these cells and molecules can be damaged over time by poor diet, lack of exercise, chronic stress, lack of quality sleep, and aging. When the brain's natural clearance system is compromised, free radicals become especially harmful.

Uncontrolled blood glucose is another biological process that contributes to Alzheimer's. The endocrine system responsible for regulating glucose levels often begins to falter as we grow older, especially when we consume a diet high in sugar and refined carbohydrates, which is stressful on our system. One dangerous consequence of glucose dysregulation is insulin resistance, which is a change in our sensitivity to insulin, a hormone that allows our bodies to regulate glucose and use it as energy. Many people are not aware that they are insulin resistant, but this disease alone can lead to significant cognitive decline and Alzheimer's disease. Once a person has progressed from insulin resistance to a diagnosis of diabetes, their risk of cognitive decline is even greater. Because the brain depends on constant balanced levels of glucose for energy, when glucose levels are out of balance, the negative effects in the brain are compounded.

Lipid dysregulation is the fourth biological process responsible for the changes associated with Alzheimer's disease. Lipids are a fatlike substance that form the building blocks of cell walls, hormones, and steroids. They are integral to cellular structure, energy storage, and all life-sustaining functions. Lipid dysregulation occurs when the body is subjected to excessive lipids, inflammation, oxidative damage, and other forms of stress on the body. In response, lipid transport and metabolism are impaired, which leads to lipids being oxidized, creating even more inflammation. We will discuss this in more detail in later chapters.

All four of these biological processes are interconnected; they all result in formation of amyloid and tangles in the brain that can lead to the progression of Alzheimer's disease. Some people may also be at increased risk for the progression of disease based on their age and their genetic makeup. But what's so incredible is that all four pathways are deeply influenced by lifestyle. The choices you make with regard to nutrition, exercise, sleep, stress, and brain stimulation can positively or negatively impact these biological processes and alter your risk of developing Alzheimer's disease.

It is important to distinguish between early-onset Alzheimer's, which occurs before age sixty, and late-onset Alzheimer's, which happens after age sixty. Early-onset Alzheimer's disease is caused by genetic mutations, such as presenilin-1 and presenilin-2, which are very rare and account for only 2–3 percent of all cases. Late-onset Alzheimer's disease is much more prevalent and is influenced by variations to other genes, such as the ApoE4 gene, which is commonly found in more than 25 percent of the population. People with the ApoE4 gene are, to some degree, predisposed to late-onset Alzheimer's disease, but the expression of this gene can be dramatically influenced by what you eat, how much you exercise, how well you sleep, and how you deal with stress. In fact, Dr. Dale Bredesen states, "Alzheimer's disease can be prevented, and in many cases its associated cognitive decline can be reversed."[3]

According to a recent report commissioned by *The Lancet* medical journal, around 35 percent of dementia cases might be prevented if people make better lifestyle choices, like exercising more and eating better. The *Lancet* report, distilling the findings of hundreds of studies, identified several factors that likely contribute to dementia risk, many of which can be controlled.[4] These include midlife obesity, physical inactivity, high blood pressure, type 2 diabetes, social isolation, and low education levels. Of course, we recognize that dementia is a complicated disease that has multiple causes and risk factors, many of which remain unknown. Nevertheless, there is increasing evidence that people, even those who inherit genes that put them at greater risk of developing Alzheimer's in later life, can improve their chances by adopting healthier lifestyle changes. Because most neurodegenerative diseases take years, if not decades to develop, researchers agree that the best time to focus on brain health is long before symptoms occur, ideally by midlife, if not before.

If all this degeneration is taking place in the brain over many years, why don't cognitive symptoms appear earlier? How is the brain able to withstand such assault without showing signs of problems until later in life? The brain is very resilient, and fortunately for all of us, it is designed with a lot of redundancy. With eighty to ninety billion neurons and nearly a quadrillion connections, as well as overlapping arteries that supply multiple regions with nutrition and oxygen, the human brain has a remarkable ability to withstand stress. It can work around neurons and parts of the brain that have literally been destroyed by plaques, inflammation, and oxidation. If it takes a hit in the form of a stroke, for example, other parts of the brain can work to offset the injury. The brain is also capable of regenerating some cells, though that capacity is limited, particularly the older we get.

In Alzheimer's patients, cognitive symptoms of the disease emerge only after there is so much damage that the brain's innate resiliency can no longer compensate. That is the biggest challenge with treating Alzheimer's disease: we only become aware of the disease once the damage is considerable.

CHAPTER TWO

The Stages and Types of Dementia

*D*r. Alois Alzheimer observed in his now-famous patient, Auguste Deter, some of the classic symptoms of advanced Alzheimer's: paranoia, outbursts, confusion, and withdrawal. In the majority of cases, the earliest symptom of Alzheimer's is difficulty with short-term memory, like forgetting what someone told you that day, or asking someone the same thing over and over. People with early signs of this disease often have trouble with numbers and keeping track of their bills. They may lose track of things and place them in unusual places. And they may start to withdraw from hobbies and social activities as their memory becomes more impaired. Over time, the disease progresses into mood swings, disorientation, difficulty with language, and the inability to carry out basic activities like bathing and putting on clothes. By definition, a person has developed dementia when he or she has difficulty with one or more daily activities, such as driving, taking medications, making phone calls, cooking, and finances.

The Seven Stages of Alzheimer's Disease

Dr. Barry Reisberg of New York University developed a method for breaking the progression of Alzheimer's disease into seven stages.[5] This framework has been adopted by a number of healthcare providers, as well as the Alzheimer's Association.

The common denominator for all stages of Alzheimer's and other forms of dementia is anxiety. Even people in the early stages experience significant anxiety because they fear further decline. Though the development and speed of the disease are unique to each individual, Alzheimer's generally progresses through each of these seven stages.

Stage 1. *No impairment. Preclinical. This stage can last 1–5 years or more.*
A person in this stage has no impairment, no memory disorder or defective thinking, but amyloid plaques and tau tangles—the "debris" caused by lifestyle choices and other stressors—may be accumulating in the brain. There may also be inflammation, vascular changes, and atrophy in certain parts of the brain, but not enough to cause symptoms.

Individuals at this stage can experience significant benefits from making lifestyle changes. Proper nutrition will slow down the inflammatory, oxidative, and vascular damage that may have already started. Exercise will help regrow neuron connections and increase blood flow to the brain. Good food choices and regular exercise will reduce insulin resistance. Stress reduction can allow the brain to heal itself, and improved sleep can help detoxify and restore the brain's function. Brain stimulation helps maintain good cognitive abilities.

Stage 2. *Very mild decline. Can last 20 years or more. Some mild memory changes begin to emerge in stage 2.*
At stage 2, a person can still do everything they've always done: finances, driving, and work responsibilities are not yet affected, and family members haven't noticed any significant changes. The person may notice minor memory problems or lose things around the house, although not to the point that the memory loss can easily be distinguished from normal age-related memory loss. The person will still do well on memory tests, and the disease is unlikely to be detected by loved ones or physicians.

This early stage can last up to twenty years before symptoms worsen. Individuals with mild decline will experience the same benefits from lifestyle changes as preclinical patients. Many individuals at this stage are able to reverse their symptoms if lifestyle change is implemented early on.

Stage 3. *Mild cognitive impairment (MCI). Lasts 1-5 years.*
At this stage, family members and friends may begin to notice cognitive problems. Perfor-

mance on memory tests is affected, and physicians will be able to detect impaired cognitive function. People in stage 3 will have difficulty in many areas, including:

- finding the right word during conversations
- organizing and planning
- remembering names of new acquaintances

People with stage 3 Alzheimer's may also frequently lose personal possessions, including valuables. A person's friends and family members may begin to notice changes in memory and thinking in this stage. The individual may deny the changes or claim they are only experiencing mild, short-term memory problems. Finding the right word, planning and organizing, and visuospatial skills like judging distance and determining color tend to present difficulties. Individuals with mild cognitive impairment will experience many of the benefits from lifestyle changes as in stages 1 and 2.

Stage 4. *Mild to moderate dementia. Lasts 2–3 years.*

A person with stage 4 may become anxious, aggressive, or withdrawn from challenging situations. Clear-cut symptoms of the disease are apparent. People with stage 4 of Alzheimer's disease:

- have decreased knowledge of current events
- have difficulty with simple arithmetic
- have poor short-term memory (may not recall what they ate for breakfast, for example)
- may forget details about their life histories

They have a hard time remembering what they did over the last week. Short-term recall is significantly affected. In the doctor's office, a person at this stage will fail to recall a list of five words. They begin having difficulty with one or more daily activities, like cooking or taking their medications.

A formal Alzheimer's diagnosis is most often made by a physician during stage 4.

This stage is somewhat troublesome because most patients are still in denial and want to maintain control of their daily lives.

Patients with mild to moderate dementia can still benefit from the plan in this book to help slow progression of the disease. Stress management is especially important for reducing anxiety, which is present for so many of these patients. Getting proper sleep is also important.

It is vital that these patients have as much social interaction as possible, as it has been observed that patients who aren't actively engaged with those around them will decline at a faster pace. It is also critical that these patients be kept safe. These patients should not cook for themselves as they might forget to turn the stove off. Driving privileges are usually taken away, and steps should be taken to protect these patients from falls.

Stage 5. *Moderate to severe dementia. Lasts 2–3 years.*
These patients can no longer survive without help from others. Confusion is pronounced; they often forget their home address, their phone number, names of more distant family members like grandchildren, where they went to school, time of year, and place. They may know their own name and that of their spouse and children. Anxiety in this stage often manifests as frustration and anger.

During the fifth stage of Alzheimer's, people begin to need help with many day-to-day activities. People in stage 5 of the disease may experience:
- difficulty dressing appropriately
- inability to recall simple details about themselves, such as their own phone number
- significant confusion

On the other hand, people in stage 5 maintain functionality. They typically can still bathe and toilet independently. They also usually still know their family members and some detail about their personal histories, especially their childhood and youth.

Stage 5 often lasts 1–2 years. It is important to try to reduce sources of anxiety as much as possible for these patients. They also benefit from cognitive and social activities. Regular exercise is very important. Alzheimer's patients in stages 5 and 6 have three times the risk of falls and hip fractures. There is much evidence that maintaining muscle strength and balance through exercise significantly reduces the chance of injury, and even increases cognitive health.

Stage 6. *Severe dementia. Lasts 2–3 years.*

Patients in stage 6 are unable to do any daily activities and are mostly unaware of their surroundings. Professional care is needed. Patients are confused, unaware of their surroundings, and experience major personality changes: sometimes aggression emerges, and other times a person completely withdraws. Sleep cycles are affected by an inability to tell night from day.

People in the sixth stage of Alzheimer's need constant supervision and frequently require professional care, such as skilled nursing and full-time caregivers. Symptoms include:

- confusion or unawareness of environment and surroundings
- sometimes forgetting spouse's name
- inability to remember most details of personal history
- loss of bladder and bowel control
- major personality changes and potential behavior problems

People in this stage may not recognize close family members. Some patients suffer from Capgras syndrome, believing that a familiar person is an imposter. Sleep cycles are also severely affected. Wandering can occur during this stage, so again, keeping the patient safe is of utmost importance.

Patients with severe dementia can still benefit from a good nutritional plan, although they will need help with feeding themselves. Exercise, stress management, and good sleep can still be beneficial to these patients.

Stage 7. *Very severe decline. The final stage of dementia. Lasts 1–2 years.*
Patients at this stage need help with all daily activities. They may become unresponsive. They often refuse to eat. They have difficulty with walking and often lose control of urine or bowel movements.

This is the final stage of Alzheimer's. Because the disease is a terminal illness, people in stage 7 are nearing death. They lose the ability to communicate or respond to their environment, and to walk. While they may still be able to utter words and phrases, they have no insight into their condition, and need assistance with all activities of daily living. In the final phase of Alzheimer's, people may lose their ability to swallow as the brain loses its ability to tell the body what to do.

Different Types of Dementia

Dementia is a general term used to describe severe changes in the brain that cause memory loss. These changes also make it difficult for people to perform basic daily activities and recognize faces. In many people, dementia causes changes in behavior and personality. In general, there are ten types of dementia.

Alzheimer's disease. Alzheimer's disease is the most common type of dementia. Between 60 and 80 percent of cases of dementia are caused by this disease, according to the Alzheimer's Association. Alzheimer's disease is characterized by brain cell death. As the disease progresses, people experience confusion and mood changes. They also have trouble speaking and walking. Older adults are more likely to develop Alzheimer's. About 2–3 percent of cases of Alzheimer's are early-onset Alzheimer's, occurring in people in their forties or fifties.

Vascular dementia. The second most common type of dementia is vascular dementia. It's caused by a lack of blood flow to the brain. Vascular dementia can happen as you age and can be related to atherosclerotic disease or stroke. Symptoms of vascular dementia can appear slowly or suddenly, depending on what's causing it. Confusion and disorientation are common early signs. Later, people with vascular dementia have trouble completing tasks or concentrating for long periods of time. Vascular dementia can cause vision problems and sometimes hallucinations.

Dementia with Lewy bodies. Dementia with Lewy bodies, also known as Lewy body dementia, is caused by protein deposits in nerve cells. These deposits interrupt chemical messages in the brain and cause memory loss and disorientation. People with this type of dementia also experience visual hallucinations and have trouble falling asleep at night, or may fall asleep unexpectedly during the day. They also might faint or become lost or disoriented. Dementia with Lewy bodies shares many symptoms with Parkinson's and Alzheimer's diseases. For example, many people develop trembling in their hands, have trouble walking, and feel weak.

Parkinson's disease. Many people with advanced Parkinson's disease develop dementia. Early signs of this type of dementia are problems with reasoning and judgment. For example, a person with Parkinson's disease dementia might have trouble understanding visual information or remembering how to do simple daily tasks. They may even have confusing or frightening hallucinations. This type of dementia can also cause a person to be irritable. Many people become depressed or paranoid as the disease progresses. Others have trouble speaking, and might forget words or get lost during a conversation.

Frontotemporal dementia. Frontotemporal dementia, also known as Pick's disease, is a name used to describe several types of dementia, all with one thing in common: They affect the front and side parts of the brain, the areas that control language and behavior. Frontotemporal dementia affects people as young as forty-five years old. Although scientists don't know what causes it, it does run in families, and its patients have mutations in certain genes, according to the Alzheimer's Society. This dementia causes compulsive behavior, as well as loss of inhibitions and motivation. It also causes problems with speech, including forgetting the meaning of common words.

Creutzfeldt-Jakob disease. Creutzfeldt-Jakob disease (CJD) is one of the rarest forms of dementia. Only one in a million people is diagnosed with it every year, according to the Alzheimer's Association. CJD progresses very quickly, and people often die within a year of diagnosis. Symptoms of CJD are similar to other forms of dementia. Some people experience agitation, while others suffer from depression. Confusion and loss of memory are also common. CJD affects the body as well, causing twitching and muscle stiffness.

Wernicke-Korsakoff syndrome. Wernicke's disease, or Wernicke's encephalopathy, is caused by a lack of vitamin B1, which leads to bleeding in the lower sections of the brain. Wernicke's disease can cause physical symptoms, like double vision and a loss of muscle coordination. At a certain point, the physical symptoms of untreated Wernicke's disease tend to decrease, and the signs of Korsakoff syndrome start to appear.

Korsakoff syndrome is a memory disorder caused by advanced Wernicke's disease. People with Korsakoff syndrome may have trouble:

- processing information
- learning new skills
- remembering things

The two conditions are linked and are usually grouped together as one condition, known as Wernicke-Korsakoff syndrome. While it's technically not a form of dementia, symptoms are similar to dementia, and it's often classified with dementia. Sometimes people with Wernicke-Korsakoff syndrome make up information to fill in the gaps in their memories without realizing what they're doing.

Wernicke-Korsakoff syndrome can be a result of malnutrition or chronic infections. However, the most common cause for this vitamin deficiency is alcoholism.

Normal pressure hydrocephalus. Normal pressure hydrocephalus (NPH) causes a person's body to build up excess fluid in the brain's ventricles. The ventricles are fluid-filled spaces designed to cushion the brain and spinal cord; they rely on just the right amount of fluid to work properly. When fluid builds up excessively, it places extra pressure on the brain. This can cause damage that leads to dementia symptoms. According to Johns Hopkins Medicine, an estimated 5 percent of dementia cases are due to NPH. Some of the potential causes of NPH include:

- injury
- bleeding
- infection
- brain tumor
- previous brain surgeries

However, sometimes doctors don't know the cause of NPH.

Symptoms include:

- poor balance
- forgetfulness
- changes in mood
- depression
- frequent falls
- loss of bowel or bladder control

Early medical intervention can prevent additional brain damage. Normal pressure hydrocephalus can sometimes be cured with surgery.

Mixed dementia. Mixed dementia indicates that a person has more than one type of dementia. Mixed dementia is very common, with the most common combination being vascular dementia and Alzheimer's. According to the Jersey Alzheimer's Association, up to 45 percent of people with dementia have mixed dementia but don't know it. Mixed dementia can cause different symptoms in different people. Some people experience memory loss and disorientation first, while others have behavior and mood changes. Most people with mixed dementia will have difficulty speaking and walking as the disease progresses.

Huntington's disease. Huntington's disease is a genetic condition that causes dementia. Two types exist: juvenile and adult-onset. The juvenile form is rarer and causes symptoms in childhood or adolescence. The adult form typically first causes symptoms when a person is in their thirties or forties. The condition causes a premature breakdown of the brain's nerve cells, which can lead to dementia as well as impaired movement. Symptoms associated with Huntington's disease include impaired movements, such as jerking, difficulty walking, and trouble swallowing. Dementia symptoms include:

- difficulty focusing on tasks
- impulse-control problems
- trouble speaking clearly
- difficulty learning new things

Other Causes of Dementia

Many diseases can cause dementia in their later stages. For example, people with multiple sclerosis can develop dementia. It's also possible for those with HIV to develop cognitive impairment and dementia, especially if they're not taking antiviral medications.

CHAPTER THREE

Can Alzheimer's Be Prevented?

The Pursuit of a Medical Cure

Today, the pursuit of a youthful mind is a multibillion-dollar industry. Sellers of vitamins, herbal supplements, and tonics claim that they have the secret to slowing the aging process while making us feel years younger and giving us the promise of a sharper mind. So, is there a magic cure for Alzheimer's disease? Is there a miracle pill that can promote brain health and youthfulness to everyone who takes it?

Probably not. Since the 1980s, scientists and clinicians have focused on treating the late stage of the disease process. And though hundreds of millions of dollars have been spent on countless experimental drugs, the progression of Alzheimer's disease has not improved. In some cases, the drugs have actually made the disease worse.

Out of over 240 experimental Alzheimer's drugs tested by the Food and Drug Administration over the past fifteen years, only one, memantine, has been approved (in 2003), and its overall effect on the disease has been disappointing at best. Memantine, also known as Namenda, works by inhibiting the transmission of excess glutamate, a neurotransmitter. Glutamate is released in excess by brain cells damaged by Alzheimer's disease, creating toxic effects, so blocking this seems like a good idea. Unfortunately, memantine may also inhibit the very neurotransmission critical to memory formation, and it does nothing to halt the progression of the disease.

One class of drugs called cholinesterase inhibitors (i.e., Aricept and Exelon) was designed to keep a particular enzyme called cholinesterase from destroying acetylcholine, a key chemical in the brain that acts as a neurotransmitter. Neurotransmitters are chemicals in the brain that carry signals from one cell to another, which allows the brain to store memories, to think and to feel, to move and perform its wide range of functions. The science behind these medicines was solid. In Alzheimer's disease, there is a marked reduction in acetylcholine. Therefore, if you block the enzyme cholinesterase, which breaks down acetylcholine, more of the neurotransmitter will remain in the synapses between brain cells, allowing the brain to function better. Although the rationale for these drugs is clear, blocking the breakdown of acetylcholine does not turn out to affect the cause or progression of Alzheimer's disease. In addition, these drugs have side effects like nausea, vomiting, diarrhea, and drowsiness that make taking them sometimes unpleasant.

In general, medications have proven ineffective at curing or stopping Alzheimer's. Furthermore, it doesn't look like there are any new promising drugs on the horizon aimed at treating the disease once the diagnosis has been made. In fact, one pharmaceutical company, Pfizer, Inc., recently announced that it was pulling out of Alzheimer's drug research altogether.

But according to a recent wave of scientific studies, we have more control over our cognitive health than was commonly known. We can take certain steps, ideally earlier than later, to live a healthier lifestyle and protect our hearts, our bodies, and our brains.

Stopping Disease in Its Earliest Stages

Fortunately, scientists around the world have started to do more work—research and clinical trials—around the earlier stage of the disease process known as mild cognitive impairment, or MCI. Not all patients with MCI will go on to develop Alzheimer's disease. But we know—through the work of Dr. Reisa Sperling at Johns Hopkins and others—that more than 15 percent of patients with MCI will go on to develop Alzheimer's disease each year.

However, we believe that even this stage of the disease process may be too late to try to stop it. We now know that at this stage of MCI, some 50–70 percent of key neurons have already been lost from patients' memory networks. If we are truly going to change the course of this disease, we are going to have to go back even further in the disease process, to the preclinical stage. This stage of the disease occurs *before* there are any noticeable memory changes. The problem is that this stage is very hard to recognize. It looks like normal aging. To recognize this disease process in its earliest stages, we will need to discover biomarkers that could identify patients on a trajectory toward MCI and Alzheimer's long before any clinical symptoms are noticeable.

This idea isn't new. In the mid-1990s, scientists observed that beta-amyloid and tau, the two common proteins that spread through the brains of those with Alzheimer's disease, also appear in spinal fluid, the colorless liquid enveloping the brain and spinal cord. (The only way to obtain this fluid is by puncturing the base of a person's spinal cord with a two-inch needle.) Researchers found that the levels of beta-amyloid and tau differed between healthy people and those with Alzheimer's: beta-amyloid was reduced in the spinal fluid of Alzheimer's patients, while tau was increased. We think this is because beta-amyloid becomes trapped in plaques inside the brain, while tau oozes out of the brain as neurons slowly fall apart. It has been shown that this can happen *20–30 years before symptoms begin*. These spinal-fluid studies can be very accurate in predicting Alzheimer's disease, but they are painful and ultimately not very helpful in developing treatment plans.

Other studies, like positron emission tomography, or PET amyloid imaging, has been used in some cases to help with early detection of this disease. Those with amyloid pathology as shown on PET imaging studies are five times more likely to develop Alzheimer's disease than those who show no signs of such pathology. But these studies are costly, and they haven't been very reliable in diagnosing the extent of disease nor helpful in developing treatment plans. Many patients who show changes on PET amyloid imaging studies have no symptoms at all. And some patients with severe Alzheimer's disease can have normal imaging studies.

So for most of our patients, we don't recommend a spinal tap to assess levels of beta-amyloid or tau. Nor do we routinely send patients to the radiology department for PET amyloid imaging studies. We do, however, recommend that each of our patients learns all they can about their own health as well as their family histories. We strongly encourage our patients to get an annual physical, including extensive lab work and genetic studies, if indicated. We recommend that our patients understand how nutrition and exercise can influence their overall health and brain function throughout the course of their lives.

After years of clinical practice, we now know that the lifestyle choices we make every day can have a profound effect on the overall health of the brain. We may not be getting the exercise we need to rid the brain of toxic amyloid. In addition, many of us aren't getting the deep sleep we need to clear amyloid from the brain and support learning and memory. Ineffective stress management and lack of brain stimulation contribute to cognitive impairment. Many of the conveniences of modern life can significantly increase the risk of brain toxicity and cognitive decline. For example, processed foods, high in sugar and saturated fats, are known to be toxic for the brain.

By making informed decisions about the foods you eat and the amount of exercise and sleep you get—simple choices you make each and every day—you can actually slow the aging process and improve your brain health. You can reduce the amount of inflammation in your body, regain your energy, improve your memory, begin to reverse the process of cardiovascular disease, and increase your overall health.

Women and Alzheimer's

Because women make up nearly two-thirds of patients with Alzheimer's disease in the United States, it is worth considering their unique potential risk factors. One in six women develop Alzheimer's after age sixty-five, while for men the chances are only one in eleven. Women in their sixties are more likely to develop Alzheimer's in their lifetime than breast cancer.

"Women age faster in their forties," said Dr. Lisa Mosconi, who studies brain images of women, at a women's health summit in 2017. She theorizes that the loss of estrogen makes the brain more vulnerable to diseases like Alzheimer's, and that women's brains age faster than men's. Dr. Dale Bredesen contends that there is an epidemic of early neurocognitive disease in women; he suggests that a cognitive evaluation should be standard as women enter their forties, just as we are all expected to have a colonoscopy when we turn fifty.

Scientists used to believe that the reason behind the prevalence of Alzheimer's among women was simply that they live longer than men, but now researchers are exploring other potential reasons: lifestyle, genetics, biology, and hormones.

In particular, researchers are exploring whether hormonal changes related to menopause may affect the development of Alzheimer's disease. Studies have shown that when estrogen production declines during menopause, the brain's metabolism appears to slow down, and it becomes less efficient. About 60 percent of women report a kind of "brain fog" when going through menopause.[6] In a study including 117 females, women in the first year of menopause performed significantly worse than women in other stages of life on verbal learning, verbal memory, motor function, and attention / working memory.[7] However, the brain seems to adapt from these changes in hormones (estrogen, progesterone, follicle stimulating hormone, and luteinizing hormone) that swing wildly during the time when a woman goes through menopause.

While some women breeze through menopause with no issues, others have more trouble. It's important to understand treatment options available and how to optimize your own body's potential. We recommend talking with your physician about menopause and your own risk factors, to determine whether hormonal replacement therapy with bioidentical hormones—hormones that are chemically the same as those the body produces—may be right for you.

You have control over at least six modifiable risk factors: midlife obesity, hypertension, diabetes, smoking, depression, and insomnia. Improvements to these factors through the lifestyle recommendations of this book can dramatically reduce your risk of heart disease and Alzheimer's disease.

Beth came to us at age fifty-eight with progressive memory loss. Her mother had died of Alzheimer's disease at age seventy-five, and she was very concerned about her own symptoms. Beth had a demanding job that required her to prepare data reports and present in front of her colleagues on a regular basis. As her symptoms progressed, she found herself becoming much more anxious about these presentations and found the work she'd once enjoyed to be "overwhelming at times." When she read a book, she would often have to reread sections that she'd just finished because she couldn't remember what she'd read. She also had trouble navigating roads that had once been familiar to her. The icing on the cake was when she couldn't remember her husband's phone number.

Our exam revealed a very pleasant but slightly anxious woman. She was a little overweight, with a body mass index of 26 (normal is 18.5–24.9). Her blood pressure was also a little elevated, at 140/88. When we got her lab work, we found that she had elevated glucose and high cholesterol, and she also had a gene that could potentially increase her risk for Alzheimer's disease: ApoE 3/4. Her levels of estrogen and progesterone were noticeably low, consistent with a postmenopausal female, as were her levels of thyroid and vitamin D (10 ng/mL, with normal being 30–100 ng/mL). It should be noted that vitamin D can actually be classified as a hormone rather than a vitamin. It is involved in almost every aspect of the body, from strengthening your bones to improving your memory and helping your immune system.

Because she was so sleepy, and her husband complained of her snoring, we also performed a sleep apnea study with a home-sleep-study device. Beth tested positive for moderate sleep apnea, which was appropriately treated.

We immediately focused on Beth's diet and exercise and put her on our diet plan along with a daily exercise regimen. She noted an immediate improvement in the way she felt and said that she no longer wanted to "take a nap" in the middle of her board meetings. We also tackled her low vitamin D and low hormone levels with vitamin D supplements and bioidentical hormonal supplements. After just three months, Beth noticed a significant improvement in all her symptoms. She was able to enjoy her work again, and her presentations were much less stressful. Most notably, her level of concentration seemed to be much better.

CHAPTER FOUR

Inflammation

*Instead of different treatments for heart disease, Alzheimer's,
and colon cancer, there might be a single inflammation-reducing
remedy that would prevent all three.*
—*Time* magazine, February 23, 2004

Let food be thy medicine, and let medicine be thy food.
—Hippocrates

*H*ippocrates, who lived from 470 to 370 BCE, is considered the father of Western medicine. His discoveries 2,500 years ago led him to advocate for the healing powers of food long before the first scientific evidence was produced. He recognized that food is not simply a tangible object to satiate hunger or relieve boredom; it is the substance that fuels our bodies and feeds our minds, maximizing performance, endurance, and longevity. Food can be a potent healer—or it can be poison.

Many of our patients suffer from a variety of inflammatory diseases: arthritis, tendonitis, lupus, vasculitis, and psoriasis, to name a few. Each of these life-changing diseases is caused by too much inflammation in the body.

Under normal circumstances, inflammation, which is part of the immune system's reaction to wounds or infection, helps the body heal itself. The body has the ability to increase circulation and boost the activity of the immune system at sites of injury and infection. When you cut your finger, for example, blood vessels near the cut expand. That clears the way for the white blood cells to destroy any bacteria that sneak in through the cut. The white blood cells also begin to mend the damaged skin by ordering in new cells to seal the cut. By the time the signs of inflammation—heat, soreness, and swelling—kick in, the wound is well on its way to healing.

Even obesity is considered a form of inflammation of the fat cells. When we gain weight, we don't create new fat cells (that number stays fairly constant from childhood). Instead, weight gain is observed when fat cells become inflamed and enlarged, storing many of the toxins we ingest daily through the foods we eat.

If the process of inflammation persists, the body can become chronically inflamed, causing a host of inflammatory disorders. Certain diseases, such as lupus, rheumatoid arthritis, psoriasis, Graves' disease, and fibromyalgia, emerge when the immune system flips on and refuses to turn off. Inflammation may also be at the root of some of our deadliest diseases, including heart disease, diabetes, cancer, and Alzheimer's disease.

In October 2018, researchers at Boston University School of Medicine found a link between chronic inflammation and the risk for Alzheimer's disease. They summarized, "While it is widely shown that possessing the ApoE4 gene is the major genetic risk factor of Alzheimer's disease (AD), not all ApoE4 carriers develop AD. For the first time, researchers have shown that ApoE4 linked with chronic inflammation dramatically increases the risk for Alzheimer's disease. This chronic inflammation can be detected by sequential measurements of C-reactive protein, a common clinical test which can be done routinely in a clinical setting."[8] Using data from the Framingham Heart Study, which includes more than three thousand human subjects, the researchers studied patients with the ApoE4 gene and those with and without chronic low-grade inflammation as defined by sequential C-reactive protein measurements. They found ApoE4 carriers *with* chronic low-grade inflammation were at greater risk for onset of dementia and Alzheimer's disease, as compared to ApoE4 carriers *without* inflammation. If chronic low-grade inflammation can be decreased among ApoE4 carriers, the difference in Alzheimer's risk between ApoE4 carriers and non-ApoE4 might also significantly decrease.

We now know that inflammation in the brain is one of the primary causes of Alzheimer's disease. A recent article in *Scientific American* noted that many studies done in the past few years are pointing toward the conclusion that both Alzheimer's and Parkinson's may be the results of neuroinflammation, in which the brain's immune system has gotten out of whack.[9] The exact process remains unknown. In some cases, the spark that starts the disease process might be some kind of insult—perhaps a passing virus, gut microbe, or long-dormant infection. Or maybe in some people, simply getting older, adding some pounds, or suffering too much stress could trigger inflammation that starts a cascade of harmful events.

To better understand how chronic inflammation can lead to diseases like Alzheimer's dementia and heart disease, it's important to know how the gut wall functions and how the foods we ingest every day can influence these processes. Your intestines are lined with a layer of mucosal cells, called enterocytes, which are locked tightly together to prevent harmful organisms and toxins from entering your body. Immune cells (specialized white blood cells) are positioned all along this lining and are very important in maintaining the integrity of this wall. These immune cells are like soldiers guarding the walls of your intestines; under normal circumstances, they prevent toxins, viruses, bacteria, and other organisms from entering our bodies and causing an inflammatory response.

Your stomach acids, enzymes, and normal gut flora work to break down the food you eat into amino acids, fatty acids, and sugar molecules. And when all is working normally, your mucosal cells pass these necessary molecules through and keep out all the bad stuff. But if this defensive mucosal barrier gets worn down, it can allow toxic compounds to enter, causing an inflammation cascade that is bad for your health. This is the definition of "leaky gut," also known as intestinal permeability, which is the major cause of many of the common diseases associated with aging. In fact, as Dr. Steven Gundry describes in his book *The Longevity Paradox*, "It's the gradual breakdown of this barrier that accelerates the aging process."[10]

The major hormones that control inflammation are called prostaglandins. Some are pro-inflammatory, meaning they produce inflammation, while others are anti-inflammatory and inhibit inflammation. The body synthesizes these hormones from many of the foods we eat. Depending on your diet, the body can create inflammation, or it can reduce the inflammatory process. Unfortunately, most Americans consume thirty times more of the foods that produce inflammatory prostaglandins than those that produce anti-inflammatory ones.

Scientists have learned that inflammation and chronic disease can be the result of a lack of the right bacterial population, or microbiome, in your gut, along with a leaky gut that allows bacteria and other toxic particles to pass through the intestinal border. By eating the right foods, you can dramatically reduce the amount of inflammation in your body and strengthen your mucosal barrier. If, however, you eat a lot of foods that cause this mucosal barrier to break down, your levels of inflammation can become toxic. A diet high in trans-fatty acids, such as stick margarine and processed foods, for example, will result in more inflammatory agents.

At our practice, we are asked every day about processed foods. What are they and why are they bad for you? By definition, a processed food is a food item that has had a series of mechanical or chemical operations performed on it to change or preserve it. Most processed foods are those that typically come in a box or bag, and contain more than one item on the list of ingredients. For most of us, it's not realistic to avoid all processed foods. In fact, some processed foods may even be somewhat healthy for us, like precooked whole grains, Greek yogurt, frozen vegetables, and canned beans. But if the "food" or ingredient can only be made in a lab or through a chemical process, like high-fructose corn syrup, hydrogenated oil, soy protein isolate, or aspartame, then consider it a highly processed food, and don't eat it.

If, on the other hand, the foods you eat are consistent with those proposed in the *Healthy Living for a Sharper Mind* plan, your body will begin to create hormones that have anti-inflammatory effects. You will begin to see your inflamed joints, skin, and arteries return to normal. Your body will become more balanced, and as a result, you will begin to feel and look younger. In addition, the amount of neuro-inflammation in your brain will decrease.

CHAPTER FIVE

Vascular Disease and Dementia

*T*he vascular system delivers blood, oxygen, and nutrients throughout our bodies, through arteries and veins. Vascular disease is an inflammatory condition that affects these arteries and veins, potentially limiting blood flow to parts of the body that are affected. This process can lead to injury and cell death in those areas. When vascular disease occurs in the heart, it can result in a myocardial infarction, or heart attack. When it affects the brain, it can result in a cerebrovascular attack, or stroke. Diseases of the vascular system—heart attacks, strokes, and hypertension—account for the majority of deaths in the United States. Common causes of vascular disease are:

Atherosclerosis. An inflammatory disease that results in a buildup of fatty deposits and narrowing of the arteries over a period of time.

Inflammation. Inflamed arteries are narrower and less efficient.

Blood clots. Some blood clots are beneficial, like when you cut yourself and the clotting of the blood prevents further bleeding. However, blood clots can also form inside arteries in the body, preventing blood flow. In the brain, for instance, this can lead to a stroke.

Trauma. A blow or multiple blows to the body can cause clots and other trauma to the vascular system.

Genetics. Certain vascular diseases, like hereditary hemorrhagic telangiectasia, can be inherited.

Each of us experiences atherosclerosis, or hardening of the arteries, as we get older. This happens over time when the smooth, elastic inner lining of the blood vessels becomes hard and begins to crack. Through these cracks can seep cholesterol, calcium, platelets, and fibrin, which can then accumulate, causing an atheroma, or plaque. Over time, more material is deposited, narrowing the artery, causing inflammation to the arteries, and reducing blood flow to the area of the body where the plaque is deposited. If this plaque reaches a dangerous level—closing off 80 percent or more of the artery—a blood clot can get stuck in the narrow passageway and obstruct blood flow. If this happens in the brain, the sudden total blockage of the artery, known as a thrombosis, or stroke, causes a portion of the brain fed by that artery to die, resulting in damage to the brain or death.

When plaque buildup happens in the arteries around the heart, it is called ischemic heart disease, which can lead to heart attack. Narrowing of the arteries to the brain can lead to transient ischemic attacks of the brain, or strokes. This understanding of vascular disease and the brain has led to the development of powerful clot-buster medications, such as tPA, that have saved the lives of many patients with strokes.

It is vital to your overall health that you work to reduce your risk factors for vascular disease. *The Healthy Living for a Sharper Mind* plan works because of its dramatic effect in lowering your risk for these vascular diseases, including dementia, heart disease, and stroke.

More than two thousand people in the United States die each day from vascular disease, namely heart attacks and strokes. Until the early 1990s, experts believed that heart disease, specifically atherosclerosis, or hardening of the arteries, was a progression of sticky cholesterol plaque built up on smooth artery walls, causing the arterial passageways to narrow. But it is now known that this model of vascular disease, wherein excess cholesterol is the culprit, is not the complete story for most heart attacks and strokes.

The Role of Inflammation in Vascular Disease

Physicians now recognize that inflammation is just as important a risk factor as cholesterol for cardiovascular disease and stroke, especially considering that up to one-half of people with known vascular disease have normal cholesterol levels.

People with obesity, diabetes, and metabolic syndrome have a much higher incidence of vascular disease. Why? High blood sugar, triglycerides, and insulin underlie a silent inflammation of the endothelium, the single layer of cells that lines the body's fifty thousand miles of blood vessels. This inflammation is not only responsible for most vascular diseases, but for most chronic diseases, including Alzheimer's and aging itself.

Arteries are normally elastic, multilayered vessels that carry oxygen to all parts of the body. As we age, however, arteries can become inflamed and less elastic, allowing damage to the vessel. This happens when LDL (bad) cholesterol seeps through the tissue layers of the vessel and sticks to the inside of the artery wall, causing damage to that site. The body then triggers an inflammatory response to contain the damage, and the artery swells, constricting blood flow to that part of the body. Over time, this causes the arteries to become less elastic, and the process of atherosclerosis, or hardening of the arteries, begins. So inflammation is directly involved with the vascular system throughout the body. Reducing levels of inflammation in the body can prevent most vascular disease, including heart attacks, strokes, and yes, even dementia.

The Role of Cholesterol in Vascular Health

What exactly is cholesterol? A common misconception is that cholesterol is the same as fat in the diet. Cholesterol is actually a waxy substance in the blood that is used for many of the body's functions.

Cholesterol serves as the building material for many sex hormones, such as estrogen and testosterone, as well as adrenal hormones, such as cortisone. It is important as well in the production of vitamin D, which helps keep bones strong by utilizing calcium.

Bile acids are also made from cholesterol, which help the body digest fats in the diet by breaking them down and secreting them into the small intestine as bile. Finally, cholesterol is a key component of glands in the skin that help protect the body from dehydration and irritation.

In order to produce cholesterol, the liver breaks down fats and carbohydrates through a process called fatty oxidation. However, when too many fats are consumed in one's diet, the body has a difficult time getting rid of the excess, and fats build up in various cells and tissues.

Diets high in saturated fats (like those found in fatty cuts of beef, butter, and cheese) and carbohydrates with a high glycemic index (such as bagels, instant oatmeal, corn flakes, and pretzels) lead to increased production of cholesterol and fatty acids. Other causes of elevated cholesterol include obesity, smoking, lack of exercise, and heredity. Certain health conditions may also increase a person's risk for high cholesterol. Alcohol abuse, diabetes, kidney disease, liver disease, and an underactive thyroid gland can all contribute to elevated cholesterol levels.

The Role of Triglycerides

High triglycerides are the result of overeating, especially eating too many refined sugars and carbohydrates with a high glycemic index, like those found in white rice, pineapple, and white bread. Like elevated cholesterol, high serum triglycerides are associated with increased risk of vascular disease.

The Role of Lipoproteins

Triglycerides and cholesterol move through the blood together in protein-coated droplets called lipoproteins. These lipoproteins are manufactured in the liver, and are the transport vehicles used to carry lipids to and from cells in the body. When fat enters the bloodstream after a meal, it is taken up by a class of lipoproteins called high-density lipoproteins, or HDL. HDL is the "good cholesterol" that carries triglycerides and choles-terol to the liver. The liver then metabolizes these lipids, sending them out to other parts of the body, or eliminating them in bile.

Lipids carried from the liver to other parts of the body are delivered in another class of transport vehicles called LDL, or low-density lipoproteins. LDL is often labeled "bad cholesterol" because it carries cholesterol and triglycerides from the liver to other parts of the body, such as the arteries, leading to atherosclerosis. High levels of LDL and low levels of HDL lead to atherosclerosis and increased risk of heart attack and stroke.

Clinicians have discovered that it's not just the absolute number of LDL and HDL particles, but also the size of the particles that is important. Advanced lipid studies, such as those done through NMR and Lipomed testing, can show seven sizes of LDL particles and five sizes of HDL particles. In general, bigger particles of lipids are better. If your body has more small particles, your risk for heart disease and stroke increases significantly, because when LDL particles are small, they can easily squeeze beneath the blood vessel endothelium linings, narrowing the passageways with a buildup of plaque. This fatty plaque can eventually lead to heart attack and stroke.

Measuring Cholesterol

Cholesterol is measured in milligrams per deciliter of blood (mg/dL). If your total cholesterol level is 200 or more, it's considered high, and your risk of heart attack and stroke is greater. In general, a person who has a total cholesterol level of 240 mg/dL has twice the risk of heart attack a person whose cholesterol level is 200 mg/dL. Knowing your total blood cholesterol level is an important first step in determining your risk for heart disease and stroke. However, a critical second step is knowing your HDL level.

HDL cholesterol that is less than 50 mg/dL is considered low. Low HDL cholesterol puts you at high risk for heart disease. Smoking, being overweight, and leading a sedentary lifestyle can all result in lower HDL cholesterol. If you have low HDL cholesterol, you can help raise it by:

- not smoking
- losing weight (or maintaining a healthy weight)
- being physically active for at least thirty to sixty minutes a day most days of the week
- eating a heart-healthy diet that emphasizes more vegetables and less sugar

LDL levels can have a dramatic impact on your risk of heart disease and stroke. The lower your LDL cholesterol, the lower your risk. LDL can sometimes be a better predictor of total risk of heart disease than total cholesterol. In general, the optimal LDL cholesterol level is less than 100.

Treatment of high cholesterol levels is a lifelong journey. Work with your doctor throughout your life to make sure your risk factors for chronic disease, such as high LDL cholesterol, hypertension, and elevated blood sugar, are minimized. In addition to the dietary and lifestyle modifications outlined in this book, your doctor may recommend medication to help lower your cholesterol, such as statins. But no matter what medications you may take, diet, exercise, and a healthy lifestyle are crucial in reducing your risk of heart disease and stroke.

CHAPTER SIX

Diabetes and Alzheimer's Disease

*R*esearchers have discovered that there is a link between a sugar-insulin imbalance and Alzheimer's disease. People with type 2 diabetes have a significantly increased risk of Alzheimer's over those who do not have diabetes. Two of the greatest threats to your brain come from too much inflammation and an imbalance of glucose and insulin. Both these threats can essentially be neutralized by diet.

Excess weight takes a toll on memory and cognitive function. Most people don't realize that their bulging bellies are literally causing their brains to shrink. And they don't realize that their high-fat, high-sugar diets are significantly contributing to their "brain fog" and lack of concentration. Being overweight not only takes a toll on our hearts, our bodies, and our brains, but it also raises the risk of developing prediabetes, metabolic syndrome, and type 2 diabetes, all of which significantly increase the risk of dementia.

Prediabetes, or impaired glucose tolerance, occurs when blood sugar is high but not high enough to meet the threshold for diabetes. It is often the first hint of increased glucose intolerance, a sign that your body is becoming unable to regulate glucose levels in the blood, and it affects an estimated eighty-five million Americans, according to the American Diabetes Association.

Metabolic syndrome is defined as a combination of central obesity (belly fat) and two or more of the following: a triglyceride level of more than 150 mg/dL; an HDL level of less than 40 mg/dL in men, or less than 50 mg/dL in women; a blood pressure of 130/85 or higher or previously diagnosed hypertension; a fasting glucose level of more than 100 mg/dL or previously diagnosed type 2 diabetes. Metabolic syndrome significantly increases your risk of developing coronary artery disease, stroke, and type 2 diabetes.

Type 2 diabetes is a condition in which the body either doesn't produce enough insulin, the hormone that helps regulate blood sugar levels, or the body's cells have become resistant to insulin. Either way, the result is elevated sugar levels, which can cause damage to blood vessels, our hearts, our kidneys, our eyes, and our brains. The Centers for Disease Control and Prevention (CDC) estimates that type 2 diabetes affects more than twenty-five million Americans, or 8.3 percent of the population.

As with each of these diseases, the importance of nutrition cannot be overstated. When you eat, the pancreas responds to the amount of glucose in your food, releasing insulin into the bloodstream. This insulin, under normal circumstances, enables the body's cells to use sugar as an essential source of energy. The pancreas is designed to regulate levels of glucose in our systems by secreting insulin in response to the amount of glucose and sugar in the foods we eat.

The pancreas, however, was not designed to handle the amount of sugar that is present in today's carbohydrate-loaded diet. Eventually the pancreas loses its ability to keep up with the increased demand of the body. As more and more insulin secretion is needed to maintain normal glucose levels, the process of prediabetes begins.

Scientists and clinicians have known for decades about the dangers of consuming the amount of refined sugar found in the typical American diet. In his 1976 bestseller *Sugar Blues*, William Dufty observed the profound negative effect of refined sugar as it was introduced to entire nations. His research made a strong case for the link between refined-sugar consumption and diabetes, as well as other diseases such as cardiovascular disease and stroke.

Some would even argue that refined sugar should be added to the "hazardous to your health" priority list (along with cigarettes and drugs). This is especially relevant when you relate the increase in diseases, like diabetes and heart disease, to eating too many refined carbohydrates, like those found in white flour, white rice, and soft drinks. These foods can spike your blood sugar quickly, which makes it more difficult for your pancreas to release enough insulin to cope with the spike.

As stated above, diabetes occurs when the body either cannot provide enough insulin, or the cells become resistant to insulin. A person with type 2 diabetes must limit their consumption of carbohydrates, take medication to reduce the amount of unabsorbed glucose in their system, or start injection insulin in order to control their blood glucose. If not diagnosed and properly controlled, diabetes can lead to heart disease, kidney failure, and blindness, among other complications.

The bottom line is that too much blood sugar can damage the cells in your brain. If you are diabetic, controlling your blood glucose levels should be your top health priority. Frequent monitoring of your blood glucose, regular visits to your doctor to check your A1C (an average blood sugar number for the previous three months), a healthy diet, exercise, and stress reduction (stress can raise the amount of sugar in your system) can all make your body healthier. In fact, in the early stages of diabetes, the disease process can be stopped and even reversed through proper diet and exercise.

By following the *Healthy Living for a Sharper Mind* plan, you will learn to reduce your intake of refined carbohydrates, embrace fiber-rich carbohydrates that do not raise your blood sugar, lower your levels of insulin, and ultimately, reduce the amount of inflammation in your body.

CHAPTER SEVEN

Obesity and Dementia

A friend of mine told me about her training session at the gym one day. Her trainer made her do walking lunges up and down the gym. She was huffing and puffing, really struggling, and glad when she came to the finish line. Then Ray, her trainer, handed her two fifteen-pound dumbbells, and said, "Do it again." Now she had an extra thirty pounds to carry while she was doing her lunges. It was even more of a struggle.

When she returned, her trainer said, "Imagine how hard it is to carry an extra thirty pounds around all the time?"

Now that was a motivator for working out!

In a world of smartphones, video games, binge-watching Netflix, and super-sized junk food, it's no surprise that weight problems are afflicting us all, with data now suggesting that heavy children are more likely to become heavy adults. The percentage of obese children and adolescents has more than doubled since the early 1970s. Obese children not only have a difficult time losing weight as adults, they also become increasingly susceptible to a host of diseases. One clear example is the recent evidence that type 2 diabetes is occurring more frequently among younger patients.

The former US surgeon general Regina M. Benjamin, MD, MBA, stated in 2010 that "the high incidence of obesity among young people is the greatest threat to public health today." It foreshadows a maturing generation plagued by high blood pressure, heart disease, complications of diabetes, and a range of other chronic conditions associated with extra pounds.

You can clearly see from recent population studies that America is gaining weight. In 1986, the average American adult male weighed 181 pounds. He now weighs 196 pounds. The average American woman used to weigh 152 pounds, and now weighs 169 pounds. Average heights did not change.

Almost 40 percent of the US population is considered obese, according to the CDC, while 71.6 percent of the population age twenty and over is considered overweight (which includes the obese). So the majority of the population is struggling with their weight. We use body mass index, BMI, to determine if a person is in the normal range, overweight, or obese. The official definition of overweight is a BMI of 25 to 30, while a BMI over 30 indicates obesity. To calculate your BMI:

BMI = weight (in pounds) ÷ height (in inches squared) × 703

Or you can refer to a BMI chart (see next page).

BMI is more strongly associated with body fat than any other indicator of weight and height. The diagnosis of being overweight is typically made when a person's BMI is greater than 25. An individual with a BMI of 25 to 27 has mild obesity (about 20 percent overweight), which is generally believed to carry moderate health risks. A BMI of 30 or higher is considered obese. The higher the BMI, the greater the risk of developing health problems. People with BMIs of 25 to 34.9 and a waist size greater than 40 inches for men and 35 inches for women are considered at especially high risk for health problems.

If your BMI is under 25, keep it there. If your BMI is higher than 25, you may be overweight and at increased risk for heart disease, diabetes, cancer, and high blood pressure. According to some studies, a BMI of 30 and above increases the risk of death from any cause by 50–150 percent!

If you are overweight, we invite you to use the *Healthy Living for a Sharper Mind* plan to help you shed the extra pounds and maintain a slimmer, healthier body for years to come. You will learn how to lose weight safely and easily—and keep it off. Losing weight is not simply a matter of counting calories; it is a combination of making healthy choices on a daily basis and increasing your physical activity.

BODY MASS INDEX (BMI) CHART

Weight

ft/in	cm	90	100	110	120	130	140	150	160	170	180	190	200	210	220	230	240	250	260	270	280	290
(lbs)	(kgs)	41	45	50	54	59	64	68	72	77	82	86	91	95	100	104	109	113	118	122	127	132
4 ft 8 in	142.2	20	22	25	27	29	31	34	36	38	40	43	45	47	49	52	54	56	58	61	63	65
4 ft 9 in	144.7	19	22	24	26	28	30	32	35	37	39	41	43	45	48	50	52	54	56	58	61	63
4 ft 10 in	147.3	19	21	23	25	27	29	31	33	36	38	40	42	44	46	48	50	52	54	56	59	61
4 ft 11 in	149.8	18	20	22	24	26	28	30	32	34	36	38	40	42	44	46	48	51	53	55	57	59
5 ft 0 in	152.4	18	20	21	23	25	27	29	31	33	35	37	39	41	43	45	47	49	51	53	55	57
5 ft 1 in	154.9	17	19	21	23	25	26	28	30	32	34	36	38	40	42	43	45	47	49	51	53	55
5 ft 2 in	157.4	16	18	20	22	24	26	27	29	31	33	35	37	38	40	42	44	46	48	49	51	53
5 ft 3 in	160.0	16	18	19	21	23	25	27	28	30	32	34	35	37	39	41	43	44	46	48	50	51
5 ft 4 in	162.5	15	17	19	21	22	24	26	27	29	31	33	34	36	38	39	41	43	45	46	48	50
5 ft 5 in	165.1	15	17	18	20	22	23	25	27	28	30	32	33	35	37	38	40	42	43	45	47	48
5 ft 6 in	167.6	15	16	18	19	21	23	24	26	27	29	31	32	34	36	37	39	40	42	44	45	47
5 ft 7 in	170.1	14	16	17	19	20	22	24	25	27	28	30	31	33	34	36	38	39	41	42	44	45
5 ft 8 in	172.7	14	15	17	18	20	21	23	24	26	27	29	30	32	33	35	37	38	40	41	43	44
5 ft 9 in	175.2	13	15	16	18	19	21	22	24	25	27	28	30	31	33	34	35	37	38	40	41	43
5 ft 10 in	177.8	13	14	16	17	19	20	22	23	24	26	27	29	30	32	33	34	36	37	39	40	42
5 ft 11 in	180.3	13	14	15	17	18	20	21	22	24	25	27	28	29	31	32	33	35	36	38	39	40
6 ft 0 in	182.8	12	14	15	16	18	19	20	22	23	24	26	27	28	30	31	33	34	35	37	38	39
6 ft 1 in	185.4	12	13	15	16	17	18	20	21	22	24	25	26	28	29	30	32	33	34	36	37	38
6 ft 2 in	187.9	12	13	14	16	17	18	19	21	22	23	24	26	27	28	30	31	32	33	35	36	37
6 ft 3 in	190.5	11	13	14	15	16	18	19	20	21	23	24	25	26	28	29	30	31	33	34	35	36
6 ft 4 in	193.0	11	12	13	15	16	17	18	19	21	22	23	24	26	27	28	29	30	32	33	34	35
6 ft 5 in	195.5	11	12	13	14	15	17	18	19	20	21	23	24	25	26	27	28	30	31	32	33	34
6 ft 6 in	198.1	10	12	13	14	15	16	17	18	20	21	22	23	24	25	27	28	29	30	31	32	34
6 ft 7 in	200.6	10	11	12	14	15	16	17	18	19	20	21	23	24	25	26	27	28	29	30	32	33
6 ft 8 in	203.2	10	11	12	13	14	16	17	18	19	20	21	22	23	24	25	26	27	29	30	31	32
6 ft 9 in	205.7	10	11	12	13	14	15	16	17	18	19	20	21	24	24	25	26	27	28	29	30	31
6 ft 10 in	208.2	9	11	12	13	14	15	16	17	18	19	20	21	22	23	24	25	26	27	28	29	30
6 ft 11 in	210.8	9	10	11	12	13	14	15	16	17	18	19	20	21	22	23	25	26	27	28	29	30

Underweight   Healthy   Overweight   Obese   Extremely Obese

Obesity is considered by some to be as bad as smoking as a contributor to inflammation in the brain. Increased body weight is a factor in the onset and severity of many diseases, including hypertension, coronary heart disease, certain cancers, and Alzheimer's disease. Other illnesses related to obesity are sleep apnea, gall bladder disease, degenerative arthritis, and infertility. Obesity is a major factor in adult-onset, or type 2 diabetes. Degenerative arthritis can be caused by obesity: extra weight places stress on the knees, hips, back, and ankles, and bones and joints bear the brunt of it.

Weight loss is an essential part of treatment for many chronic diseases. In most cases, even a modest weight loss (5–10 percent) can result in dramatic improvement of many illnesses. The CDC estimates that 71.6 percent of Americans are overweight or obese, resulting in more than 400,000 preventable deaths each year.

Since BMI is often not a good indicator of a person's muscle mass versus fat, and is not a good measure of obesity in the elderly, it's important to note another number: a waist-to-hip ratio (WHR). To calculate this, you take your waist measurement and divide it by your hip measurement. Women with a rate higher than 0.85 and men with a rate higher than 0.90 are considered centrally obese (also known as the "beer belly" look, or being "apple-shaped") and therefore have a higher rate of Alzheimer's. Central obesity is associated with an increased risk of cognitive decline. Being big around the middle is very unhealthy, not just for your brain, but for your heart, your liver, and your pancreas. Weight carried in this area is called visceral fat, because it covers the viscera—the organs in the main cavity of the body, especially the abdomen—and produces hormones and chemicals that increase inflammation and cause insulin resistance.

Dead Weight

Perhaps nowhere is the issue of obesity in America more clearly illustrated than in the coffin business. The typical coffins of one specialty coffin-manufacturing company are now doublewides—44 inches across—compared with 24 inches for a standard model. With extra bracing, and reinforced hinges and handles, these coffins are designed to handle 700 pounds of "dead weight." Over the past several years, sales at the company have increased 20 percent annually.

CHAPTER EIGHT

Sleep and Its Effect on Brain Health

We have learned a great deal about sleep and its role in our health in recent years. Sleep science and the sleep industry has become a billion-dollar business. It seems like every other person seems to be tracking their sleep through apps or devices, or they have special pillows, lights, sheets, beds, blinds, eyeshades—all in the pursuit of the elusive perfect night's sleep. But can you recall the last time you woke up feeling refreshed, not needing a cup of coffee to get you going? If the answer is no, you're not alone. Two-thirds of adults fail to obtain the recommended eight hours of sleep their brains need each night.

The CDC calls insufficient sleep a public health epidemic, noting that fifty to seventy million Americans suffer from a sleep disorder. Lack of quality sleep presents a real danger to our brains. Without adequate rest, your body and brain suffer; prolonged periods of poor sleep are likely doing more damage than we ever imagined. Serious sleep disorders like sleep apnea have been shown to actually shrink the hippocampus and cerebral cortex, wither blood vessels, and erode brain tissue. Even poor sleep habits like habitually staying up late and waking up early, and not getting enough sleep each night may be harmful to your brain.

According to Dr. Matthew Walker's book *Why We Sleep*, "Insufficient sleep is a key lifestyle factor determining whether or not you will develop Alzheimer's disease."[12] Sleeping less than six or seven hours a night on a routine basis can dramatically suppress your immune system and double your risk of getting cancer. Inadequate sleep can disrupt blood sugar levels, contribute to cardiovascular disease, and set you on a path to congestive heart failure and even stroke.

Your brain needs sleep, seven to eight hours of good restful sleep, to rid itself of all the buildup of "trash" it has accumulated throughout the day. The space between brain cells, called the extracellular space, expands during sleep, allowing more calcium and magnesium ions to flow through. This is thought to flush out cellular debris, including beta-amyloid, one of the proteins associated with impaired brain function and Alzheimer's disease. In fact, losing just one night of sleep has been shown to lead to an increase in amyloid. So, a good night's sleep is associated with reduced formation of amyloid and can also help repair and support brain cells.

The University of Rochester Medical Center scientists who made this discovery named this function of the brain the "glymphatic system," because it functions a lot like the body's lymphatic system in removing waste from the body, and is operated by the brain's glial cells.

Scientists didn't just identify the glymphatic system—a groundbreaking discovery in and of itself—they also found that the glymphatic system goes into overdrive during sleep. When we go into deep sleep, the scientists discovered, the glymphatic system becomes ten times more active in clearing waste from the brain. This is some of the most compelling research yet to show the importance of healthy sleep in long-term brain health. If you sleep poorly or go without sufficient sleep on a regular basis, you risk missing out on the full effects of this cleansing process.

Healthy sleep unfolds in a predictable pattern, cycling through periods that are categorized as non-rapid eye movement (NREM) and rapid eye movement (REM). NREM accounts for about 75 percent of your night's sleep and occurs in stages, during which you fall progressively deeper into slumber. During these stages, your breathing and heart rate slow down, your body temperature drops, and your brain waves change from the short spikes of an awake brain to longer, slower waves. During your deepest and most restful stages of sleep, your blood pressure drops and your muscles relax.

NREM is followed by REM sleep, an active brain period during which dreaming occurs. Brain waves in REM sleep are short and choppy, similar to those in the awake brain. The body, on the other hand, is inactive, except for the eyes, which dart back and forth under closed eyelids. People cycle through NREM and REM sleep all night, with REM stages becoming longer as the night progresses. As morning approaches, our cortisol level rises, helping to make us more alert when awakening. Increased stress can also cause higher levels of cortisol, which may be responsible for waking us up too early and causing us to have a hard time getting back to sleep.

In recent years, we've begun to discover just how important sleep is for learning, memory, and behavior. Sleep, it turns out, helps us consolidate the information we receive while awake.[13] In particular, the slow brain-wave activity of certain stages of sleep seems to aid in remembering key facts and information, while REM sleep may help us process procedural memory.[14] Fragmented or poor-quality sleep, then, may interrupt or hinder the consolidation of memories for long-term storage! A good night's sleep is an important way to improve your memory.

More than eighteen million Americans are estimated to have sleep apnea, a potentially serious disorder that can lessen the quality of your sleep, as well as contribute to high blood pressure, heart disease, mood disorders, memory issues, and drowsy driving / car accidents. With sleep apnea, breathing repeatedly stops and starts during sleep. Risk factors include age and obesity; sleep apnea is more common in men. Other risk factors include sleep postures, like sleeping on your back, which can make your throat muscles relax, reducing the amount of oxygen that goes to your brain. Snoring and labored breathing during sleep as well as daytime drowsiness can all be signs of sleep apnea. If a partner or roommate or family member has complained about your snoring, or you wake up and gasp for air, or if you never feel fully rested even on the weekends, you may want to talk to your doctor about doing a sleep study to see if you have sleep apnea. It should be noted that there are several very effective treatments for sleep apnea including weight loss, specially-made dental appliances, and continuous positive airway pressure (CPAP) machines. If you think you may have sleep apnea, we recommend you talk to your doctor and see if a sleep study is right for you.

Menopause can also disturb sleep because of hot flashes and nighttime awakenings. Talk to your doctor if hot flashes are an issue in your life. Sleep is a vital part of our health, and not something we can shrug off or power through without it affecting our health in a major way. When we pay attention to our sleep, it will pay dividends in lifelong good health.

CHAPTER NINE

Concussions and Toxins

*I*n the search for what causes Alzheimer's disease, researchers have found there may be influences in addition to physical and lifestyle factors. External elements may also play a role in triggering Alzheimer's and other forms of dementia. From head injuries to the insecticide DDT and even secondhand smoke, there are elements at play in our daily lives that affect our brain health in ways we're only just beginning to understand.

Concussions

A lot of attention is currently being paid to the long-term effects of concussions on NFL players. In 2005, researchers published the first confirmed case of chronic traumatic encephalopathy (CTE) in an NFL player. Since then, further research has been done to examine the link between multiple concussions and CTE. In a study published in the *Journal of the American Medical Association* in 2017, a study of 111 deceased NFL players found that a shocking 99 percent had CTE!

CTE is a degenerative brain disease that has been identified in professional athletes, military veterans, and others who have a history of repeated head trauma. The disease is caused when the tau protein forms clumps that spread through the brain, killing brain cells (sound familiar?). Symptoms include changes in mood and behavior, aggression, depression, and paranoia. As the disease progresses, patients may experience memory loss, confusion, and impaired judgment.

While CTE is not Alzheimer's disease, there have been instances where both are present in the same patient. The study of the effects of concussions and brain injuries is important to understanding brain health over time, especially considering new research that links head injuries to an increased risk of developing Alzheimer's later in life.

Of course, concussions aren't limited to NFL players and other professional athletes. Defined as a mild traumatic brain injury caused by a bump, blow, or jolt to the head or body, a concussion can happen to anyone. The damage occurs when injury causes the brain to move rapidly inside the skull.

While there are reports of anywhere between 1.6 and 3.8 million sports-related concussions each year, an even greater number of people, more than 8 million, visit the emergency department every year for falls. According to the Brain Trauma Foundation, falls are the leading cause of traumatic brain injury, followed by car accidents, getting hit by or colliding with an object, or suffering an assault.

The number of reported concussions from falls and other accidents might be a low indicator of how many people suffer from concussions for two reasons. First, many times doctors will use "head injury" as the diagnostic term in the file, rather than "concussion." Also, there is no way of knowing how many non-sports-related head injuries do not receive medical care. Without coaches and trainers around to recognize the symptoms of a concussion, a person might not even know to seek treatment.

Concussions can lead to immediate symptoms of headache, nausea, fatigue, confusion or memory problems, and sleep disturbances. These are all short-term symptoms. But research has found there might be long-term effects as well.

In research done at Boston University Medical Center, doctors found that multiple concussions can accelerate Alzheimer's disease-related brain atrophy and cognitive decline in people who are at genetic risk for the condition. When combined with genetic factors, concussions may be associated with accelerated cortical thickness and memory decline in Alzheimer's-relevant areas.[15]

This research complements the findings at the University of Texas Southwestern in

Dallas, where researchers found that people who experienced a traumatic brain injury with loss of consciousness for at least five minutes were diagnosed with Alzheimer's disease an average of two and a half years earlier than their peers.

While much more research needs to be done for us to fully understand the link between brain injury and Alzheimer's, it seems certain that some relationship exists between the two.

Toxins

Toxins in our environment might also play a role in how this disease manifests. Every day, we're exposed to chemicals in our environment, some knowingly, and some without our knowledge. From the foods we eat to secondhand smoke, we take in a variety of harmful chemicals in our daily lives.

Pesticides are one of the heavy hitters when it comes to causing harmful medical effects in humans. For many years, we've been aware of the harmful side effects of the pesticide DDT, and in 1972, the use of this substance was banned in the United States. At that time it was shown to be linked to higher incidences of breast cancer, and since then has also been linked to higher rates of miscarriage, male infertility, and liver damage.

Now scientists have found that DDT may also be a contributing factor in Alzheimer's disease. Researchers at Rutgers University conducted blood tests on subjects with and without late-onset Alzheimer's, and found that people with the disease had levels of DDT in their blood four times greater than the control group. Interestingly, some people within the group tested had high levels of DDT but were not diagnosed with Alzheimer's.[16] Clearly, there is a link between pesticides and Alzheimer's, though the correlation is not yet well defined.

Another class of toxin we're exposed to on a regular basis is the nitrogen-based chemicals used in fertilizers. Not only are these chemicals used in agriculture, they're also widespread in the packaged food industry in the form of nitrates and nitrites, used to preserve, flavor, and color processed foods.

Sodium nitrites are added to cured meats, bacon, and sausage to help prevent bacterial growth and keep that healthy red color in the meat while it sits waiting to be purchased. Once we eat these foods, the acid in our stomach reacts with the nitrites to turn it into toxic nitrosamines, which can damage mitochondria and block insulin receptors. This in turn causes neurological damage—including, possibly, Alzheimer's.

Air pollution is another source of toxic chemicals that could be linked to Alzheimer's. Mice exposed to aerosolized nickel nanoparticles, a component of air pollution, developed amyloid plaques. Studies have also found a possible link between dementia and particulate matter, a by-product of combustion.

The harmful effects of secondhand smoke can now be linked to Alzheimer's, among many other detrimental health issues. A study by a researcher at King's College London found participants with the most severe dementia reported being subjected to high levels of secondhand smoke.[17]

CHAPTER TEN

Inflammation and Genetics—Why Inflammation Helps Us and Hurts Us

Sixty-five million years ago, life on Earth was different. These were the days of the Cretaceous period, when much of the world's current land mass was still submerged under the oceans. Although the caveman would eventually make his way up the evolutionary chain, planet Earth was dominated at this time by the dinosaur. When it comes to staying power, the hundred million years that these mega-reptiles lorded over our planet's terra firma is the longest such stretch in history—the ultimate example of terrestrial dominance. But their dominance was not to last.

The Cretaceous period ended with a very big bang: an asteroid the size of San Francisco smashed into the Yucatan Peninsula in Mexico. The collision "literally rocked the world, releasing 420 zettajoules of energy, or two million times more muscle than the largest nuclear bomb ever exploded. The resulting crater was 110 miles wide."[18] The impact was a planetary killer. Megatsunamis, massive earthquakes, global firestorms, and a deadly cascade of volcanic eruptions swallowed the earth. The sun disappeared behind a huge dust cloud—and didn't emerge for a decade. The changes to the global environment were so rapid and so extreme that the dinosaurs—the uber-dominant form of life at the time—were unable to adapt, and went extinct.

For the human species, this was very good news. Over the next hundred million years, mammals adapted to their new environment and replaced the dinosaurs as the new kings of the world. Homo sapiens evolved and have passed on their genes from one generation to the next for the past 1–2 million years. Arguably, one of the most important genes for the evolution of mankind was the ApoE gene.

ApoE Gene

The ApoE gene encodes the protein apolipoprotein E, a cholesterol carrier that is found in the brain and other organs. The ApoE gene is vital to the functioning of the body, the cardiovascular system, and the brain. Today there are several variations of this gene, but from the dawn of humankind until relatively recently, ApoE came in only one "flavor," or allele (type of gene), called epsilon 4 or ApoE4. For millions of years, therefore, our early ancestors all carried two copies of ApoE4, one inherited from each parent.

It is now known that the ApoE4 allele is strongly associated with inflammation, the very process linked to cardiovascular disease, arthritis, and many other diseases. In fact, aging itself can be linked to inflammation. Inflammation is the process that so many of us try to avoid by taking anti-inflammatories like baby aspirin or fish oil every day, or by eating foods that can have anti-inflammatory effects.

So why is it that these genes that have been present for millions of years in the evolutionary process actually promote inflammation? It's likely that they helped protect early man by promoting a robust inflammatory reaction in response to life-threatening infections. Imagine our early ancestors living on the savanna, being exposed to all sorts of pathogens, wound infections, and toxic invaders. They needed the strongest inflammatory response they could get. In terms of human evolution, ApoE4 is the oldest of the ApoE genes and was thought to protect our caveman ancestors from some of the bacteria and fungal infections they were exposed to.

Up until a couple hundred years ago, humans didn't have to worry too much about their retirement years; they had a lot more pressing fears, like not dying of disease in their youth, and not dying from war and famine. Now that we are living longer lives, however, too much inflammation can actually promote a host of chronic diseases.

Today, one in four people has this ApoE4 gene that can make them three to ten times more susceptible to developing late-onset Alzheimer's disease. If you inherit a single variant of ApoE4 from one of your parents, your risk of Alzheimer's disease can be increased by as much as 30 percent. If you inherit this gene from both your parents, your risk can be increased by 50–90 percent.

This is important: **Having the ApoE4 gene does *not* mean you will get Alzheimer's disease.** There are many ApoE4 carriers who, even at age eighty or ninety, do not have any symptoms of dementia. In fact, most people who have the ApoE4 variant never develop Alzheimer's, and more than half of the people with Alzheimer's have no copies of ApoE4 gene at all. But people with one copy of ApoE4 who do get Alzheimer's tend to get it earlier than patients with no copies of ApoE4, and people with two copies of ApoE4 who develop Alzheimer's will do so earlier still.

The ApoE protein's exact role in the development of Alzheimer's disease is unclear. Dr. Warren Strittmatter, a neurologist at Duke University, discovered a direct link between ApoE and amyloid plaque in the brain. Since then, several studies have shown that ApoE may be involved in beta-amyloid aggregation and clearance, influencing the onset of beta-amyloid deposition that is believed to contribute to Alzheimer's disease.

About 220,000 years ago the first ApoE3 gene came along. This mutation was much less inflammatory than the ApoE4 gene, and people with ApoE3 were less likely to die from cardiovascular disease and Alzheimer's. Another mutation about eighty thousand years ago brought about the ApoE2 gene. Even more recently, an ApoE1 gene has been discovered, but is extremely rare.

Today, most people carry two copies of ApoE3. This gives them a genetic risk of Alzheimer's of about 9 percent. But 25 percent of Americans, about seventy-five million people, carry a single copy of ApoE4 that they inherited from one of their parents. They have a risk of Alzheimer's disease of about 25–30 percent. Seven million Americans carry two copies of ApoE4, pushing their risk well above 50 percent for developing this disease. For people who carry one copy of ApoE4, symptoms typically begin in the late fifties or sixties; for people who carry two copies of ApoE4, symptoms can begin as early as the late forties or fifties.

Like everyone else, you have two ApoE genes, in one of the following combinations:

- ApoE 4/4. Very rare. 2 percent of the population. Increases risk of Alzheimer's by 50 percent or more.
- ApoE 3/4. 25 percent of the population. Increases your risk of Alzheimer's by 25 percent.
- ApoE 3/3. Roughly 70 percent of the population. Risk of Alzheimer's is 9 percent.
- ApoE 2/4. Risk of Alzheimer's is the same as general population, around 9 percent.
- ApoE 2/3. Risk of Alzheimer's can be reduced by as much as 10 percent as compared to the general population.
- ApoE 2/2. Risk of Alzheimer's can be reduced by as much as 20 percent as compared to the general population.

The ApoE4 variant is the number-one known genetic risk factor for late-onset Alzheimer's Disease (abbreviated LOAD), as well as for cardiovascular heart disease. A simple test of your blood or saliva will reveal your ApoE genotype; knowing your ApoE4 status can help you know what to do to lower your risk for getting Alzheimer's disease.

Family history is also a significant risk factor for Alzheimer's disease. Although the ApoE4 variant is the single strongest genetic indicator, having a first-degree relative (such as a parent or sibling) with Alzheimer's can also more than double an individual's risk of developing Alzheimer's. Individuals with a first-degree relative with Alzheimer's are at even higher risk if that relative has the ApoE4 variant.

It is important to know your family history. Understand your genetic risk for developing Alzheimer's disease and work to reduce the risk factors you can control. By understanding some of the causes of Alzheimer's disease, you can begin to address your risk factors and lower your chances of getting this disease.

Genetics Is Not Destiny

It is very important to understand that *not everybody with ApoE4 will get Alzheimer's disease*. The way the human body operates is extremely complex, and we have only identified a few of the many, many genes in our body that work together to make us unique. Since everyone is different, it's harder to figure out what exactly is going on in our bodies—what affects some might not impact others. In addition, the expression of genes can vary greatly from person to person. Our genes can switch "on" and "off" depending on their environment and our lifestyle choices.

You have the ability to affect the expression of your genes by how you manage your lifestyle choices. Everything you do—how you eat, how well you sleep, the amount of exercise you get, how you spend your free time, the quality of your relationships, and your overall stress levels—can affect the expression of your genes. Reducing the level of inflammation in your body can dramatically reduce the incidence of Alzheimer's disease, regardless of your genetic makeup.

Several important studies illustrate the role of epigenetics in the development of neurodegenerative disease. Epigenetics is the study of heritable changes in the expression of genes that do not change the DNA sequence itself. The Honolulu-Asian Aging Study found that Japanese people living in the United States have a higher prevalence of Alzheimer's than those living in Japan. There was little genetic variance among the men in this study, so the increased risk of Alzheimer's can be attributed almost solely to the epigenetic influence of poor diet, lack of exercise, and other unhealthy behaviors that are common in modern American life.

In countries like China and India, epigenetic consequences can be somewhat measured as people move away from traditional agrarian rural lifestyles and adopt more "modern" ways of living. In many of these instances, diets that are traditionally high in a wide variety of vegetables and whole foods are often traded in for more processed foods, red meat, refined sugar, and saturated fats. In addition, many of those who move to more urban environments become more sedentary, and many have more stressors in their lives. These dramatic and unfortunate lifestyle shifts can lead to changes in the expression of key genes that promote disease, often giving rise to worsening chronic diseases. China now has the world's largest diabetes epidemic, with 11.6 percent of adults developing this condition, and millions more with prediabetes. China is also ranked second for obesity, behind only the United States. As both diabetes and obesity are major risk factors for dementia, dementia is also increasing at an alarming rate in China.

Numerous studies have shown that the lifestyle choices we make every day can dramatically influence our overall health. In his best-selling book *The Blue Zones*, Dan Buettner identified five communities in the world (he could only find five) where people live measurably longer and healthier lives due to optimal nutrition, exercise, stress management, and social support. The five cities were Sardinia, Italy; Okinawa, Japan; Ikaria, Greece; Nicoya, Costa Rica; and Loma Linda, California. As Buettner explains, the nine tenets of healthy living in Blue Zones are:

- a lifestyle that involves natural movement throughout the day
- a deep sense of purpose or meaning
- skillful stress management
- avoiding overeating and eating late at night
- a primarily plant-based diet
- enjoying a drink with friends on occasion
- connection to a faith community
- living near family and finding a lifelong partner
- access to social networks that support healthy living

Buettner's groundbreaking research on behaviors common to these diverse cultures has since inspired researchers to investigate the underlying science. Cities across the world have adopted features of the Blue Zone lifestyles, such as increasing access to fruits and vegetables, volunteer opportunities, and community centers, in hopes that residents can reduce their risk of chronic disease and experience healthier and longer lives.

The bottom line is: even if your genetics seem scary—especially if you have a first-degree relative who has Alzheimer's or you have an ApoE4 gene—you have the ability to affect the expression of your genes by how well you manage your lifestyle choices.

PART II

Healthy Living for a Sharper Mind

CHAPTER ELEVEN

Comprehensive Medical Evaluation

As a primary care physician, I am asked every day by friends and family what they should do in order to stay healthy. Many of my friends approaching middle age are realizing that as they get older, it becomes harder to stay fit. It's true. After about age forty, our bodies don't work the way they did when we were younger. It takes more time to heal from an injury, our metabolism can be slower, and it is certainly harder to lose weight than it was in our twenties and thirties.

So how do we get started on the path to optimum health? One of the best things we can do is establish a good relationship with a primary care physician and get a comprehensive medical evaluation each year. Talk to your physician and work with him/her to develop a plan to make sure you are meeting your goals. Here are some of the things that we check to be sure the patients in our practice are on track to optimizing their health and living well.

Weight

Keeping your weight on track is extremely important. The epidemic of obesity and the chronic inflammation it causes to our bodies is the single biggest factor responsible for our current healthcare crisis. Check your body mass index and be sure you are in the normal range. For many of us who are even slightly overweight, losing just 10 percent of our current weight can dramatically reduce our chances of developing heart disease, Alzheimer's disease, diabetes, and even some cancers. Know what your percentage of body fat is; some scales on the market now can effectively gauge your lean mass, water, and percentage of body fat. The chart below illustrates that women typically have a higher percentage of body fat than men. As the percentage of body fat increases, the amount of silent inflammation in your body also increases. You can also measure your waistline (at the belly button) to get a good idea if you have excess body fat.

		GOOD	IDEAL
% Body Fat	Male	20%	15%
	Female	25%	20%
Waist Circumference	Male	<40 in.	< 35 in.
	Female	<35 in.	<30 in.

Blood Pressure

Your blood pressure reveals a lot about your overall health. Blood pressure is the force of blood against the artery walls. As you age, your blood pressure is more likely to rise, primarily due to your arteries becoming less elastic. Elevated blood pressure can significantly increase your risk not only for heart-related diseases, but also for cognitive impairment associated with Alzheimer's disease.

The potential role of cardiovascular health and blood pressure in dementia has been one of the surprising highlights of the Framingham Heart Study, which has followed thousands of residents of Framingham, Massachusetts, and their relatives since 1948.

The research found a 44 percent decline in the dementia rate among people age sixty and older for the period 2004–2008, compared with 1977–1983. Over that same period, the average age at which dementia was diagnosed rose from age eighty to eighty-five! Co-author Claudia Satizabal, an assistant professor at UT Health San Antonio, says the research suggests that improvements in cardiovascular health help explain the trend. And as dementia rates have fallen, the study says, so have the rates of stroke and other cardiovascular diseases. This is in large part from better blood pressure control and the wider acceptance of blood pressure medications.

You should start having your blood pressure checked once per year after age forty. With early detection, potential problems can be treated before they advance into something more serious. It has been estimated that nearly one in three Americans has high blood pressure, and many people don't know it. High blood pressure has been called the "silent killer" because it often yields no symptoms but puts us at increased risk for heart disease, stroke, and dementia.

Follow your doctor's advice and work to get your blood pressure under 120/80. If you have persistently elevated blood pressure, talk to your doctor about your options for getting your pressure under control. In patients with hypertension, blood pressure medications, such as ACE inhibitors, have been proven to reduce a person's risk of dementia and halt the progression of cognitive decline.

Eyes

Have your eyes checked. As you age, you might notice your eyesight isn't as sharp as it once was. It's important to get your eyes checked to make sure your vision is where it should be. Vision problems can pose a danger in everyday life, especially while driving. After age forty, you may start to lose sharpness in your eyes due to the lens hardening (this is natural with aging). But once you hit fifty, the symptoms can escalate, so you should have annual eye exams to make sure your vision is still up to par. Also, it's important to have a retinal screening exam. This can now be done easily in a physician's office without dilating your eyes, and can rule out early changes such as diabetic retinopathy and changes in the backs of your eyes.

Hearing

Have your hearing checked. You may be surprised to learn that hearing loss, even mild levels of loss, can increase the long-term risk of cognitive decline and dementia. Decreased hearing alone has been associated with a 9 percent increase in Alzheimer's disease. Hearing loss occurs in 32 percent of individuals over fifty-five. Evidence suggests that hearing loss continues to increase dementia risk in later life. The mechanism underlying cognitive decline associated with hearing loss is not clear. Hearing loss may add to the cognitive load of a vulnerable brain leading to changes in the brain, or it may lead to social disengagement or clinical depression, which can lead to an acceleration of cognitive decline.

EKG

An electrocardiogram, or EKG (sometimes called ECG), checks your heart activity. The EKG is used to check for signs of heart disease. Small electrode patches record your heart's electrical activity to see if there are any signs of rhythm problems with the heart. This test allows your doctor to determine how normal your heart rhythm is, see if you have poor blood flow to your heart muscle, diagnose a heart attack, and notice anything abnormal, such as a thick heart muscle. Those over fifty are at a greater risk for heart disease, so it's important to have an EKG once per year.

Cardiac Calcium Test

Developed by Dr. Arthur Agatston, author of *The South Beach Diet*, this high-resolution CT scan measures calcium plaque, or arteriosclerosis, in the vessel walls around the heart and can be a good indicator of cardiovascular health.

Carotid IMT (Intima-Media Thickness) Test

The carotid intima-media thickness (IMT) test uses ultrasound technology to measure the thickness of the carotid arteries located in the neck, where blood-flow-blocking inflammatory plaque first develops. Abnormal, premature thickening of the arterial walls is an early indicator of inflammation and vascular disease throughout the body. The thicker the arterial wall, the greater the risk for heart attack or stroke. This test is a simple, noninvasive, fifteen- to twenty-minute outpatient procedure that involves no pain, no needles, no pills, and exposes you to no radiation. During the test, you lie flat on an exam table for approximately fifteen minutes. A small amount of gel is applied to your neck, and sound beams are used to look at the thickness of your carotid arteries and for plaque formations. Ask your physician if carotid IMT testing is appropriate for you.

Blood Tests

The comprehensive metabolic panel (CMP) is a frequently ordered panel of fourteen tests that gives a healthcare provider important information about the current status of a person's metabolism, including the health of the kidneys and liver, electrolyte and acid-base balance, as well as levels of blood glucose and blood proteins. Abnormal results, and especially combinations of abnormal results, can indicate a problem that needs to be addressed. The CMP includes the following tests:

- **Glucose.** Energy source for the body; a steady supply must be available for use, and a relatively constant level of glucose must be maintained in the blood.
- **Calcium.** One of the most important minerals in the body; it is essential for the proper functioning of muscles, nerves, and the heart, and is required in blood clotting and in the formation of bones.

Proteins

- **Albumin.** A small protein produced in the liver; the major protein in our blood.
- **Total protein.** Measures albumin as well as all other proteins in the blood.

Electrolytes

- **Sodium.** Vital to normal body processes, including nerve and muscle function.
- **Potassium.** Vital to cell metabolism and muscle function.
- **CO2 (carbon dioxide, bicarbonate).** Helps to maintain the body's acid-base balance (pH).
- **Chloride.** Helps to regulate the amount of fluid in the body and maintain the acid-base balance.

Kidney Tests

- **BUN (blood urea nitrogen).** Waste product filtered out of the blood by the kidneys; conditions that affect the kidney have the potential to affect the amount of urea in the blood.
- **Creatinine.** Waste product produced in the muscles; it is filtered out of the blood by the kidneys, so blood levels are a good indication of how well the kidneys are working.

Liver Tests

- **ALP (alkaline phosphatase).** Enzyme found in the liver and other tissues, bone; elevated levels of ALP in the blood are most commonly caused by liver disease or bone disorders.
- **ALT (alanine aminotransferase, also called SGPT).** Enzyme found mostly in the cells of the liver and kidney; a useful test for detecting liver damage.
- **AST (aspartate aminotransferase, also called SGOT).** Enzyme found especially in cells in the heart and liver; also a useful test for detecting liver damage.
- **Bilirubin.** Waste product produced by the liver as it breaks down and recycles aged red blood cells.

A complete blood count (CBC) is a blood test used to evaluate your overall health and detect a wide range of disorders, including anemia, infection, and leukemia. A CBC measures several components and features of your blood, including:

- red blood cells, which carry oxygen
- white blood cells, which fight infection
- hemoglobin, the oxygen-carrying protein in red blood cells
- hematocrit, the proportion of red blood cells to the fluid component, or plasma, in your blood
- platelets, which help with blood clotting

Cholesterol Levels

Cholesterol is essential for the body to function, but at high levels, it can be dangerous. High total cholesterol (240 mg/dL or higher) in midlife increases the risk of Alzheimer's later in life by 60 percent. Even borderline-high cholesterol (200–239 mg/dL) increases the risk of dementia in old age by greater than 50 percent. Your total cholesterol levels should be at less than 200 mg/dL. A simple blood test will tell your doctor your cholesterol levels. If your levels are high, your doctor will likely recommend lifestyle changes or medications to help you live longer and healthier.

Advanced lipid studies. Elevated lipids, or hyperlipidemia, is the most modifiable risk factor leading to heart disease and stroke, yet more than 50 percent of people with "normal" lipids can have significant heart and vascular disease. Prevention of this disease includes early screening and providing the best treatment plan for each patient with disease.

Total cholesterol, HDL-C (good cholesterol), LDL-C (bad cholesterol), and triglycerides have long been considered the primary risk factors for heart disease. We now know this is not necessarily the case. In fact, traditional cholesterol testing misses up to 50 percent of people with significant cardiovascular disease. Advanced lipid testing is a tool that can dramatically improve your doctor's ability to screen you for early cardiovascular disease and provide you with the best personalized treatment plan.

What is the science behind advanced lipid testing? Just as oil and water don't mix, oil-soluble lipids—such as cholesterol and fat—don't mix with blood, which is mostly water. To do its job around the body, cholesterol has to be packaged in envelopes of protein, such as lipoproteins. Not all lipoprotein particles look or behave alike. Some are large, fluffy, and light; others are small and dense. Big, fluffy ones bounce off artery walls, but dense particles are more likely to penetrate artery walls. People who mainly have small, dense particles have *triple* the risk of coronary heart disease and stroke! Because lipoproteins are influenced by genetics, you may ask your doctor to order advanced lipid testing if you have a family history of cardiovascular disease or relatives who died early from heart attacks.

Triglyceride/High-Density Lipoprotein (HDL) Ratio

The higher your TG/HDL ratio, the higher your insulin levels are and the greater your amount of silent inflammation. A ratio of 2:1 is good and less than 1:1 is ideal. A ratio greater than 2:1 identifies you as having increased silent inflammation. It's interesting to note that the average American has a TG/HDL ratio of 3.3. Those with a ratio of 4 or more are at increased risk for type 2 diabetes.

Measuring Inflammation

There are many blood tests currently available to measure silent inflammation and dysfunction of the lining of your arteries. Make sure your doctor is checking for silent inflammation.

C-Reactive protein. CRP is produced by the liver in response to any type of inflammation. Specifically, you want to know your hs-CRP (high-sensitivity CRP). Your hs-CRP level should be below 0.9 mg/dL. If it is higher, you should work with your doctor to determine the source of the inflammation. High levels of CRP can mean increased inflammation and an increased risk for chronic disease, including cardiovascular disease and Alzheimer's disease.

The ratio of albumin to globulin in your blood (A/G ratio). Along with CRP, this is a complementary measure of inflammation and should be less than 1.8.

The ratio of omega-6 to omega-3 in your red blood cells. While both these fatty acids are important for health, omega-6s are pro-inflammatory while omega-3s are anti-inflammatory. The ratio of omega-6 to omega-3 should be less than 3 but not below 0.5.

Homocysteine. High levels of homocysteine are important contributors to heart disease and Alzheimer's disease. Any level above 6 micromoles per liter may pose a risk. Keeping your homocysteine levels optimally low requires sufficient levels of vitamins B6, B9 (folate), and B12. We recommend checking for these levels in your blood to see if you are in optimal range. When you get your blood tested for vitamin B12, you may see that the "normal" range is 200–900 pg/ml. We recommend that you have a level over 500 to be sure that you are metabolizing homocysteine optimally and reducing the levels of inflammation in your body. Many physicians also order an MMA (methylmalonic acid) test as well as a B12 test. These tests are complementary and can help determine your levels of B12. Folate levels should be in the range of 10–25. B6 levels should be 60–100.

Blood Sugar and Insulin Levels

You can be screened for prediabetes, or metabolic syndrome, a group of risk factors for myriad diseases, including heart disease and stroke. Among the causes of metabolic syndrome are being overweight, having insulin resistance, being physically inactive, and genetic factors.

Metabolic syndrome is a serious health condition. People with it have a higher risk of diseases related to fatty buildups in artery walls, such as coronary heart disease, and stroke. People with this syndrome are also more likely to develop type 2 diabetes. In recent years, this syndrome has become much more common in the United States. About 20–25 percent of adult Americans are estimated to have it. So how can you be screened for metabolic syndrome? Ask your physician to screen you for the following findings:

- increased waist circumference: over 40 inches for men, over 35 inches for women
- fasting blood triglycerides are 150 mg/dL or more
- low HDL (good) cholesterol levels (men: under 40 mg/L; women: under 50 mg/dL)
- elevated blood pressure of 130/85 mm Hg or higher, or taking medicine for high blood pressure
- fasting glucose (blood sugar) of 100 mg/dL or more
- abnormal insulin levels

If you have three or more findings from this list, you could be at risk for metabolic syndrome.

Thyroid

Optimal thyroid function is crucial for each of us. Thyroid function affects metabolic speed and many facets of the way your body functions, including your heart rate and mental sharpness. It can also impact the way you sleep, how hot or cold you feel, and how your weight is maintained. Thyroid function can easily be tested by measuring levels of free T3, free T4, and TSH (thyroid-stimulating hormone). TSH is produced by your pituitary gland and essentially instructs your thyroid to release more thyroid hormone. Thus high TSH can indicate low thyroid function. Normal levels of TSH are considered to be 0.4–4.2 microIU/l. Optimal levels of free T3 are 2.3 to 4.0 pg/ml. Optimal levels of free T4 are 1.3–1.8 mcg/dL.

Vitamins

Talk to your physician about whether a multivitamin may be right for you. Just one multivitamin per day that contains B vitamins, such as niacin and folic acid, might help protect brain tissue in some people.

Vitamin D. Vitamin D acts more like a hormone than a vitamin. Reduced vitamin D levels can be associated with everything from depressed mood to osteoporosis to heart disease to cognitive decline. Vitamin D travels through every cell in your body and is vital to your overall health. We get vitamin D when sunlight converts a cholesterol molecule, 7-dehydrocholesterol, into an inactive form of vitamin D, which is then converted into the active form. We can easily check the level of vitamin D in your system by measuring a serum level of 25-hydroxycholcalciferol; the level should typically be in the 40–80 range. Many people have low levels of vitamin D, which can easily be treated by taking a D3 supplement. You should work with your physician to see what dose is right for you.

Hormones

Scientific research indicates clear connections between declining hormones in the body and a number of diseases, including Alzheimer's. Decreasing estrogen levels in women can cause significant aging effects, such as poor brain circulation and increased levels of inflammation on the brain. Lower levels of testosterone in men can cause memory impairment and cognitive decline.

Estrogens and progesterone. In women, estrogens—estradiol, estriol, and estrone—and progesterone are essential for optimal cardiac function and brain function. A recent study by the Mayo Clinic showed that women who had their ovaries removed by age forty without hormone replacement therapy had double the risk of Alzheimer's disease of women with their ovaries intact.[19] Goal level for estradiol: 50–250 pg/ml; for progesterone: 1–20 ng/ml.

Testosterone. The sex steroid hormone testosterone is present in both females and males, but at higher concentrations in males. Goal for men: total testosterone: 500–1000 ng/dL; free testosterone: 6.5–15 ng/dL.

Cortisol. Cortisol levels can be elevated in times of stress. The goal: cortisol (usually testing in the morning as that's when they're the highest): 10–18 mcg/dL.

DHEA. Dehydroepiandrosterone (DHEA) is a naturally occurring hormone that can help slow the process of aging, and should be 250–430 mcg/dL in women and 400–500 mcg/dL in men.

More research is needed on hormonal therapies to better understand the risks and benefits as potential treatments for early cognitive decline. Bioidentical hormonal therapies, those that are most identical to those in a particular body, can be beneficial to your brain as well as your heart. Talk with your physician to decide if hormone-replacement therapy is right for you.

Metals

Zinc and copper. The balance of zinc and copper in your body is important. Blood levels of both copper and zinc should be approximately 100 mcg/dL, and the ratio should be around 1:1.

Magnesium. Magnesium is critical for brain function. Red blood cell magnesium levels should be 5.2–6.5 mg/dL.

Selenium. Selenium plays a key role in clearing free radicals from our system, and reductions in selenium have been shown to be associated with cognitive decline. Goal: Serum selenium: 110–150 ng/ml.

Heavy metals: mercury, lead, arsenic, and cadmium. These tests are not done routinely but can be very helpful in a comprehensive physical examination. Goal: mercury under 5 mcg/L; lead under 2 mcg/dL; arsenic under 7 mcg/L; cadmium under 2.5 mcg/L.

Sleep Studies

Sleep apnea is extremely common and usually goes undiagnosed. It can contribute significantly to heart disease and cognitive decline. Sleep deprivation and sleep apnea can also increase the risk of obesity, diabetes, and depression. A good night's sleep is essential for a healthy brain. Ask your doctor whether you need a study to rule out sleep apnea. This can be done easily at home with a portable sleep apnea study kit.

Cancer Screening

Colorectal. Most colorectal cancer screenings should begin at age 45—50, and you should be checked at least once every five years. If you have a family history of this type of cancer or any symptoms like bleeding, your doctor may recommend screening for colon cancer at an earlier age. As your body ages, colon cancer can become more common, so tests are imperative. Men have a one in twenty-one chance of getting the disease; for women, it's one in twenty-three.

Skin. You should have an annual skin exam looking for skin cancers, such as basal cell carcinoma, squamous cell carcinoma, and melanoma. Skin cancer can arise at any age, but after fifty years of being exposed to the sun, you should start to pay closer attention to the moles on your body. Melanoma, for example, is typically diagnosed in your early sixties, but it can show up in people much younger. Most skin cancer cases are easily treated, but melanoma can be very serious. If there are any moles on your body that seem to have changed in size, shape, or color, consult your dermatologist for a professional analysis.

Dental Health

Get a dental checkup twice a year. There is a significant relationship between gum disease and chronic inflammation, cardiac disease, even dementia. A study published in *Science Advances* in January 2019 suggests that brain and oral health are closely linked. It found that the bacteria plaque on the surface of the teeth may even spur the production of beta-amyloid proteins. Specifically, the study found that a certain type of bacteria in periodontitis (*Porphyromonas gingivalis*) was also present in the brains of people with Alzheimer's. The bottom line is that keeping your teeth clean, flossing every day, preventing periodontal disease, and seeing your dentist regularly is important.

Quantitative Neuropsychological Testing

There are many tests currently available that can evaluate your memory and your overall cognition. The simplest is the MoCA (Montreal Cognitive Assessment) test, which takes about ten minutes to administer. A normal MoCA score is 26–30; 19–25 is associated with mild cognitive impairment; 19–22 can signal dementia when associated with difficulties with activities of daily living; and scores lower than 19 reveal moderate dementia.

There are other simple tests, such as the Mini-Mental State Examination and the Self-Administered Gerocognitive Examination, which may also be helpful. There are also more extensive tests available online that can provide a more detailed analysis of brain function. Ask your physician about neurocognitive performance testing and whether it is something you should do as a baseline.

Genetic Marker Testing

Consider genetic marker testing. The ApoE4 test is an easy one and can give you an idea of your underlying risk for Alzheimer's disease and cardiovascular disease. Also, a test called DNAge can provide you with an accurate assessment of your true "epigenetic age," which takes into account the genetic factors that will determine how you age.

Flu Shot

Get a flu shot every fall, especially if you're over fifty. Those with weakened immune systems, including older people, are more likely to have serious complications from something like the flu. In some cases, the flu can lead to pneumonia, which can be very difficult to recover from in someone with a compromised immune system—it can be fatal. A flu vaccine can save your life, or at least keep you from being bedridden for a few days.

Mental evaluation

It's somewhat of a chicken-and-egg dilemma: does depression lead to Alzheimer's, or does Alzheimer's lead to depression? The answer may be a little of both. Often people diagnosed with Alzheimer's will present with depression, especially in the early and middle stages. Depression is a risk factor for dementia, and people with more symptoms of depression tend to suffer a more rapid decline in thinking and memory skills.

Either way, it's important to know the signs and symptoms of depression and talk to your doctor about treatment options. Signs of depression include:

- feelings of sadness that persist more than two weeks
- disturbances in your sleep (not able to get to sleep, or sleeping more than usual)
- fatigue
- irritability
- lack of motivation to do daily activities
- overeating or loss of appetite

Be aware that for people diagnosed with Alzheimer's, depression may present a little differently. Symptoms may come and go, or not be as severe. In addition, the cognitive impairment experienced by people with Alzheimer's may make it more difficult to communicate feelings of sadness, hopelessness, or guilt associated with depression.

Finding help is important, as treatment of depression can make significant improvements in quality of life.

Review Your Overall Health Plan

Sit down with your physician on a regular basis, assess your risk factors, and develop a plan for you to achieve your optimum health.

CHAPTER TWELVE

Sleep

"*E*arly to bed and early to rise makes a man healthy, wealthy, and wise." This proverb, made part of our common lexicon thanks to Benjamin Franklin's *Poor Richard's Almanack*, speaks a truth in its simplicity. While it is just one of many proverbs that talk about how hard work can lead to success, it also focuses on the importance of sleep and links good sleep to good health. We've come a long way in our medical research since the 1700s: we now have scientific research that validates this proverb.

During sleep, our brain is hard at work consolidating the information we absorbed while awake, which helps with learning and memory. Sleep also allows the brain to reenergize the body's cells and clear out waste. Without the proper amount of sleep, we can face myriad health issues.

It's easy enough to see the effects of lack of sleep on a daily basis. When you stay up too late binge-watching your favorite sitcom, you find yourself drowsy at work the next day and in need of coffee just to stay alert. Lack of sleep affects your energy levels, but it also affects your cognitive processes, making you feel moody or irritable and hindering your ability to remember and process information.

Tiredness is an immediate result of lack of sleep, but there are many more things sleep can impact in the body. Less than six to seven hours of sleep a night can dramatically suppress your immune system, double your risk of cancer, disrupt blood sugar levels, and contribute to cardiovascular issues. Lack of sleep also leads to an increase in beta-amyloid in the brain.

The Right Amount of Sleep

Now that you know just how important it is to get enough sleep, the question is how much sleep do you need? The answer isn't a simple one-size-fits-all, but following general guidelines and paying attention to your body's natural rhythms can help you find the magic number that fits you.

The National Sleep Foundation recommends seven to nine hours of sleep for adults ages eighteen to sixty-four, and for people over sixty-five the recommendation shifts to seven to eight hours a night. That comes with a caveat that some people might need only five to six hours of sleep, while others need as much as ten. It's hard to dictate exactly how much sleep each person needs because genetic factors and individual differences in circadian rhythms can affect sleep requirements for optimal health and physical performance.

One way to figure out how much sleep you need is to keep a sleep journal. Use it to track how many hours of sleep you get each night. Rather than just writing down "eight hours," make sure to track the actual time you went to sleep and when you woke up. You should also write down how you slept, if you slept soundly through the night or if you were up multiple times. Then keep note of how you felt during the day. After a few days, you'll start to see some correlation between how much sleep you get and how you feel each day.

For many people, just carving out time in the day to get enough hours of sleep can be a challenge. Busy schedules, demands of work, and never-ending household chores beckon continually, tempting you to stay up late or get up early to get more accomplished. Of course, stress and anxiety can lead to restless nights or an inability to go to sleep when you're tired. There may be physical issues keeping you from getting enough sleep as well, such as sleep apnea, hot flashes during menopause, or even heartburn.

Getting Better Sleep

The first step toward getting better sleep is to address any physical issues that might be keeping you up. Talk to your doctor about things like hot flashes, snoring/sleep apnea, heartburn, and stress.

There are many good wearable devices now that help you track your sleep. Some fit under your mattress; others are worn like a watch or a ring. All help track the time you're awake, the amount of REM sleep you got, the amount of deep sleep you got, and some track your resting heart rate. Many people are surprised to find out how often they awaken at night but don't remember. A more old-fashioned way to keep track, of course, is a sleep journal. Write down when you went to sleep and woke up, and whether you woke up in the middle of the night. Make note of any insomnia, or middle-of-the-night insomnia, when you wake up in the middle of the night and struggle to fall back to sleep.

Managing your stress is another way to help get better sleep, and many environmental factors and lifestyle choices can also contribute to a good night's sleep.

Pay attention to what you consume during the day. Caffeine, nicotine, and even some medications, such as inhalers, are stimulants that can keep you awake and affect your sleep. In addition to keeping you awake, studies have found that caffeine can delay the timing of your body clock, reducing the number of hours you sleep, and it can reduce the amount of deep sleep you have each night. Caffeine stays in your system anywhere from six to eight hours; nicotine, which works in the body similarly to caffeine, can stay in the system up to fourteen hours. Quitting smoking and avoiding caffeine are two ways to help improve your sleep. If you can't cut out caffeine completely, try to avoid consumption after three p.m.

You'll also want to limit alcohol consumption, as alcohol can have negative effects on sleep. Many people think a nightcap will help them get to sleep, and while you might feel drowsy after drinking a cocktail or glass of wine, alcohol is a depressant that affects the quality of your sleep later. Alcohol also reduces the melatonin in your body, a key facilitator of sleep and regulating sleep cycles. Drinking alcohol before bed blocks REM sleep, the most restorative sleep, and it can affect your circadian rhythm, causing you to wake up in the middle of the night.

Another way alcohol affects your sleep is by increasing your probability of snoring. As a depressant, alcohol intake relaxes your muscles, including those in the jaw and throat, which causes the muscles to collapse on your airway and restrict airflow.

Get regular exercise. Making a workout part of your routine is a good way to create better sleep, as one study showed that regular exercise cut in half the amount of time it took participants to fall asleep. Following a moderate aerobic exercise routine can increase the amount of short-wave sleep your body gets each night. It doesn't take much exercise to get results: at least thirty minutes of aerobic exercise per day can improve sleep habits relatively quickly.

It's important to note that while exercise can help with sleep, you don't want to work out right before going to bed. This will stimulate your endorphins and keep you awake.

Establish a sleep routine. If you often have trouble falling asleep, you might want to try creating a sleep routine. The same thing that works for babies works for adults as well. Rather than just shrugging off your clothes and hopping into bed, allow yourself time to wind down and get ready for sleep. Your sleep routine might include taking a hot bath or shower, reading or listening to music, or performing meditation. All of these can help your body relax.

You might also try progressive muscle relaxation. This is where you lie down and try to empty your mind of all your worries. Concentrate on one muscle group at a time, tightening your muscles as you breathe in and relaxing them as you breathe out. Start with your feet, move to your legs, then your arms, then your torso, and finish with tightening and relaxing your entire body.

You'll notice that our tips for a sleep routine don't include TV. The light and activity (people's voices, storylines, moving figures) from television and other screens, such as phones and tablets, impairs the secretion of melatonin and provides cognitive stimulation that keeps your brain from relaxing. One study showed a 22 percent decrease in melatonin levels in people engaged with screens in the hours before bed. Put away those screens and turn off the TV an hour or two before bedtime, and make something else a part of your regular bedtime routine.

Create a good sleep environment. The atmosphere where you sleep plays a big role in helping you get better rest. One of the first things to pay attention to is lighting. Use low wattage bedside lamps rather than bright overhead lights in your bedroom at night before going to bed. This helps signal to your body that it's time to go to sleep. The temperature should be comfortable, and a little on the cool side. Studies show between 60 and 67 degrees Fahrenheit is an optimal temperature for sleeping, and some people enjoy it even cooler. The cooler temperatures help your body release more melatonin. Also, our body temperature bottoms out right around five p.m. and rises slowly through the night, so a cool room helps keep you from waking up hot and improves sleep duration and quality.

Finally, having a comfortable bed to sleep in can help improve the quality of your sleep. If you haven't replaced your mattress in over seven years and you wake up with a bad back each morning, it might be a sign that it's your mattress that needs replacing. Your pillows should be replaced every year.

Once you've found your good sleep routine and perfect environment, make sure to follow it on a regular basis. The final key to better sleep is to try to make the time you go to bed and wake up similar from day to day. Fluctuations in sleep time can disrupt your natural circadian rhythms.

Better sleep will have you feeling more energized, will help in your cognitive performance, and will help keep you healthy. It's an easy way to take advantage of your body's natural defenses on your path to good health.

CHAPTER THIRTEEN

Exercise

*Physical fitness is not only one of the most important keys to a
healthy body, it is the basis of dynamic and creative intellectual activity.*
—John F. Kennedy

When you gain control of your body, you will gain control of your life.
—Bill Phillips, Body for Life

The human body, a magnificent machine with 206 bones and 640 muscles, is obviously meant to move, yet the muscle that probably gets the greatest workout is the *gluteus maximus*—the one we sit on.

What most people don't realize is that few lifestyle choices have as great an impact on health as physical activity. Exercise can affect our bodies and minds as dramatically as the foods we eat. That is why exercise is an essential component of the *Healthy Living for a Sharper Mind* plan. Fortunately, no matter how old you are or how long you've been inactive, it's not too late to begin a fitness program, because there is no age limit for reaping the benefits.

Why is exercise so important?

Heart health. Being active boosts high-density cholesterol and decreases unhealthy triglycerides, reducing the risk of cardiovascular disease.

Energy level. Physical activity delivers oxygen and nutrients to the body, maximizing the cardiovascular system and increasing your energy level.

Disease prevention. Regular physical activity is also shown to sharply reduce the risk of diabetes, metabolic syndrome, stroke, high blood pressure, and even dementia.

Cancer prevention. Much of current exercise research is focused on cancer prevention and treatment. Some studies indicate that those who exercise have decreased risk of developing colon and breast cancers. In addition, recurrence among breast cancer survivors may drop by half when an exercise program and healthy diet are included in treatment. Other research suggests that physical activity can also reduce the risk of endometrial and lung cancers. Dr. Lee W. Jones, associate professor and scientific director of the Duke Center for Cancer Survivorship, has found that some types of cancerous tumors grow 30–50 percent slower in mice that are exercised, as opposed to those that aren't.[20]

Weight control. If you've tried to lose weight, you know that exercise is paramount to your efforts. Exercise can also boost endurance, improve bone and muscle strength, aid in the ability to conduct daily activities, and prevent falls.

Longer life. According to the CDC, studies have shown that those who are physically active for more than 150 minutes a week have a lower risk of dying prematurely than those who are active for less than thirty minutes a week.

Better mood. What's good for the body is good for the soul. Physical activity stimulates various chemicals in the brain that improve your mood, enabling you to feel happier and more relaxed, while relieving depression and anxiety. Exercise also promotes better sleep, which can aid in the prevention of heart disease, as well as increase your level of concentration and improve your mood.

Better sex life. If that's not enough to convince you to exercise, what about your sex life? Regular physical activity can leave you feeling energized and looking better, which may have a positive effect on your sex life. What is more, physical activity can lead to enhanced arousal in women and less erectile dysfunction in men—a winning combination.

How Much Exercise Do You Need?

The US Department of Health and Human Services, the American College of Sports Medicine, and the American Heart Association agree: all adults ages eighteen to sixty-four should get 150 minutes of moderate-intensity exercise per week. This recommendation can be broken down into thirty minutes of moderate-intensity exercise five days per week, or twenty to sixty minutes of vigorous-intensity activity three days per week. Adults sixty-five and older and those with chronic conditions or physical limitations are also encouraged to exercise, but with moderate intensity under physician supervision. No matter how long you exercise, the degree of intensity is key in your journey to better health. The US Department of Health and Human Services' *Physical Activity Guidelines for Americans* has more specific recommendations:

- 150 minutes a week (approximately 20 minutes a day) of moderate-intensity aerobic (cardio) exercise (example: brisk walking), plus at least two days of anaerobic activities that work the major muscle groups (hips, legs, shoulders, back, abdomen, chest, arms), or
- 75 minutes a week (a little over ten minutes each day) of high-intensity aerobic exercise, such as jogging, plus two days of whole-body muscle-strengthening activity
- an equivalent combination of moderate and high-intensity aerobic exercise, plus two days of whole-body muscle-strengthening activities

One minute of high-intensity exercise is the equivalent of two minutes of moderate-intensity exercise: the same benefits in half the time. However, if you haven't exercised in a while, you will need to increase your level of activity slowly to avoid injury and health problems.

Ten at a Time

Don't be overwhelmed by the number 150. Break down the 150 minutes into ten-minute increments, which is easier to tackle, especially if you haven't exercised in a while. Just be sure, no matter the activity, that you are doing it in a moderate or vigorous effort. A ten-minute walk, three times a day, five days a week equals 150 minutes!

How Do You Get Started?

If you've been sitting behind a desk for years and have forgotten what it's like to feel the wind on your face and the strength of your leg muscles pushing against a bike pedal as you propel yourself around the block, you're in for a pleasant surprise. The rewards of exercise are many, as physical activity can be as enjoyable as it is beneficial. Exercise gives you a chance to unwind, enjoy the outdoors, do something completely different, connect with friends and family, or simply engage in activities that make you happy. Talk with your doctor before beginning an exercise program if you have a chronic condition, such as diabetes or heart disease. The two of you can come up with a plan that matches your abilities. Remember, any physical activity, no matter how small, is better than none.

Understand that cardiac events, such as heart attacks, are rare during physical activity, but the risk goes up when you become more active suddenly. Therefore, it is wise to start slowly and gradually increase your level of activity. Start with brisk walks before attempting jogging, or bike on a flat surface before tackling the hills. Working your way to a healthy body is simple: Find an activity you enjoy, dedicate yourself to doing it, and commit to a routine. You don't have to join a fitness center or sign up for classes. To start, all you really need is a good pair of walking shoes and thirty minutes five days a week to enjoy nature. Couple your walk with strength-training exercises two days a week, and you're well on your way. If walking doesn't excite you, find something that does. If you're miserable while exercising, you simply haven't found the right activity for you. Commit to trying a new activity or class every few weeks for several months. You're bound to come across a form of exercise you truly enjoy.

Find Your Motivation

Why do you want to exercise? The answer to this question is important because there will be days when you will not feel like moving—when you'd rather sit and read a good book or go out with your friends. Your motivation may be as frivolous as getting back into a dress or pair of pants you wore two years ago, or as serious as lowering your cholesterol or blood sugar levels. Regardless of the reason, knowing the answer will keep you on track.

If you feel more motivated with others, join a fitness center. Circuit training and spinning are often easier in groups. Register for classes: dance, yoga, Pilates, or water aerobics. Get a personal trainer to show you some moves with weights, how to use all the machines, and what the correct form is so you don't get injured. Join a team: basketball, softball, or soccer. Find a partner: tennis or golf. If sweat equity is all the motivation you need, stair climb, cycle, or run. Try to move every day. Small efforts will add up at the end of the week.

If it's your significant other who needs to exercise, ask him or her to join you when you exercise. Skip your run and suggest a long walk. Within a few weeks your partner will be walking—or running—without being asked. You may even want to use this time to learn something new together, like ballroom dancing or pickleball.

A Pound a Month

A pound of body fat equates to approximately 3,500 calories. Just two brisk twenty-minute walks a day, five days a week, burns about 695 calories. This means that without changing your diet, that you could lose over twelve pounds in a year!

Discover Your Inspiration

Getting inspired begins with shaking up your regular routine and beginning a new one, taking strides to improve your fitness habits as you go. But inspiration can come from a multitude of sources. For starters, check with your city's park and recreation department. You may be surprised by the number of activities offered, and many are inexpensive—or free. Many communities have access to clubs, groups, coaches, and teams, all designed to get you active.

Next, scan your local paper for activities. From 5K run/walk events to disc golf tournaments, you'll recognize activities you enjoy. Many events are fundraisers for diseases or social issues. Find one that raises money or awareness for a cause close to your heart. These good-karma activities will inspire you to get in shape. You are also likely to meet people with strong fitness backgrounds who may help push you to your next level.

Think about activities you enjoyed when you were young. If you ran track in high school, start jogging. If you were a swimmer, check out the local aquatics club. If you played tennis, grab a racket and head for the neighborhood court. If you don't have a hitting partner, find a backboard to practice your stroke. You'll be amazed not only at the workout you get but also how much your game will improve. Regardless of the source of inspiration, use it to help achieve your fitness goals. Change begins when you think outside your comfort zone and open yourself to new and exciting possibilities.

Set a Goal

Your ultimate fitness objective is to have a healthy body, but how do you achieve this? First, you set a goal.

Rule No. 1: Your goal must be attainable.

Rule No. 2: Your goal must be challenging.

Start small; think big. If you've decided to participate in a future 5K event, begin walking through your neighborhood or local park. Then jog for a minute and walk for a minute. As you become more comfortable, pick up the pace and add hills to your route. Soon, you will be jogging with confidence.

Once you have established an appropriate goal for your fitness level, lifestyle, and interest, you are ready to make positive changes to become more active. Little by little, you will have more energy and see noticeable improvements in your overall health and wellness. Incorporating new behaviors into your lifestyle will have a huge impact on your success.

Experts agree that if you force yourself to change your behavior for three weeks, your brain will start to release dopamine in response to the behavior you are trying to acquire. Therefore, if you skip the after-work get-together and head to the gym, in three weeks your brain will be craving a good workout rather than your favorite libation. Be realistic in setting your goal, and remember, you don't have to be perfect. If you miss a day, kick it up a notch the next day and recommit to your routine.

Attain Your Goal

Having set a realistic goal, you now need to put in the time, effort, and self-discipline necessary to attain it. An important component is addressing your interests and motivation. Continue to participate in activities you enjoy with people who inspire you. The point is to have fun while you exercise. If you need to take a break for personal reasons or injury, or simply need a rest, don't lose sight of your goal. Ultimately, an exercise routine should be such a regular part of your daily activities that you don't have to think about it—just like brushing your teeth or washing your face before bedtime. When you reach your goal, celebrate your success and then get reinspired. Try a new activity. Be on the lookout for a different group. Incorporate a more challenging set of weight-training exercises. Your body and mind will thank you.

Fitness and Nutrition

Glycogen is the body's main source of carbohydrate storage. The harder and longer you exercise, the more glycogen your body uses. Pre-exercise fuel should consist mostly of carbohydrates, which burn quickly. Examples include wheat bread with a teaspoon of almond butter, or high-fiber cereal with a banana.

After exercise, your body looks for ways to replenish glycogen. Therefore, if you exercise for more than an hour, it is important to eat a healthy snack that includes protein, carbohydrates, and fat within an hour after you finish. These include:

- apple slices with almond butter
- smoothie made with fresh fruit and low-fat yogurt
- whole-wheat bagel and bananas
- pita or carrots with hummus or avocado
- sweet potato with cinnamon
- nuts

Stay Hydrated

Water consumption before, during, and after a workout is crucial to good health. Skip the sports drinks, which contain large amounts of sugar. Unless you are working out for over an hour in intense heat and losing electrolytes, hydrating with water remains the most effective and efficient way to decrease your risk of dehydration.

Exercise Your Options

Aerobic versus Anaerobic Activity

There are two types of exercise: aerobic and anaerobic. *Aerobic* means exercising in the presence of oxygen. Aerobic exercise involves raising your heart rate enough to burn excess body fat and get your blood pumping more efficiently. Most physical therapists

Time Constraints

If finding the time to exercise is difficult, rethink your daily routine. Walk in place or use resistance bands while you're watching television. Take the stairs instead of the elevator. Get up forty-five minutes earlier (if you can do so while still maintaining a healthy amount of sleep), use part of your lunch hour to walk, or commit to half an hour of exercise after work, rather than plopping down on the sofa. Many fitness centers are open 24/7, making it easier for those with erratic schedules to find the time to exercise. Numerous videos—from yoga to Pilates, strength-training to aerobics— have been created for home use. Workout videos are convenient and inexpensive alternatives to joining a gym or studio. Find an activity you enjoy and commit to it at least three times a week.

Regardless of the activity you choose, create an appropriate space in your home to do it. Make sure the area has ample room to move your arms and legs and is set apart from distractions.

recommend exercising to the degree that your heart rate increases to some percentage of its maximum. A good approximation of your maximum heart rate is 220 minus your age. Therefore, if you are 50, an intense aerobic workout should get your heartbeat to a maximum of 170 beats per minute.

The latest research indicates that the maximum benefits for increased longevity and improved health occur when you expend more than 2,000 calories per week during exercise. Walking one hour per day can burn more than 300 calories. If you walk six hours per week, less than an hour per day, you can greatly improve your health and dramatically reduce your overall risk of premature death.

Higher-intensity exercises, like jogging, burns about twice as many calories per hour as walking. Therefore, in order to get the same cardiovascular benefits as walking every day, you only need to jog two to three hours per week. The higher the intensity of exercise, the more hormonal and cardiovascular benefits you will achieve. The exercise intensity that induces the most improved balance of hormones and endorphins is between 60 and 70 percent of your maximum heart rate.

In contrast to *aerobic*, *anaerobic* means without oxygen. Anaerobic exercise uses muscles at high intensity for short periods of time, building and maintaining muscle strength. If the intensity of the anaerobic workout is high enough, it causes the body to release specific hormones that can significantly improve overall well-being. These hormones can work immediately to reduce body fat and gain lean muscle mass. Anaerobic exercise also increases bone density and strength, reshapes the body, and can increase your metabolism by building muscle mass.

While our brains know how old we are, our muscle cells rely on heart and muscle activity. When they're not activated by regular aerobic exercise and strength training, muscle cells deteriorate and lose fortitude. When you exercise, no matter your age, your body responds in a youthful manner. The more muscles are stimulated, the more they regenerate and prepare for more rigorous exercise. Studies on inactive older adults participating in resistance training showed not only a slowing of age-related muscle disintegration but an actual reversal in the aging of the muscle at gene level. Weight-lifting, sprinting, jumping, and resistance training are examples of anaerobic activity. Strength training is the most effective type of anaerobic exercise.

Cardiovascular Activities: What Counts?

Cardiovascular activities increase your breathing and heart rate. According to the CDC, all types of activity count—from yoga to pushing a lawn mower—as long as you are doing it at a moderate to vigorous intensity for at least ten minutes. Light daily activities such as laundry or shopping aren't considered cardiovascular in nature, because they don't increase your heart rate. Moderate-intensity cardiovascular activity means that you are working hard enough to raise your heart rate and break a sweat. You can talk during the activity but can't sing the words to your favorite song. High-intensity cardiovascular activity means that you're breathing hard and fast, and your heart rate is very accelerated. If you are working at this level, you won't be able to say more than a few words without pausing for a breath.

Moderate-Intensity Exercise

- ballroom dancing
- bicycling on level ground (slower than 10 mph)
- gardening
- pushing a lawn mower
- tennis (doubles)
- walking briskly (3 mph or faster)
- water aerobics
- yoga (a good beginner's yoga is hatha)

High-Intensity Exercise

- aerobic dancing
- bicycling or spinning (faster than 10 mph)
- elliptical or stair climber
- heavy gardening
- hiking uphill
- jumping rope
- swimming laps
- team sports such as basketball or soccer
- tennis (singles)

How Many Calories Am I Burning?

If you're trying to lose weight, it is important to know how many calories you are burning during your workout. The number of calories burned depends on whether you're male or female, how much you weigh, and your BMI. The numbers below are estimates of the number of calories burned in thirty minutes.

Activity	Calories burned in 30 min.
Aerobics, low impact	200
Baseball	105
Basketball	230
Bicycling, moderate pace	135
Bicycling, mountain	237
Dancing, moderate effort	200
Disc golf	84
Elliptical trainer, serious effort	390
Golf, walk with clubs	120
Jogging, moderate pace	240
Pilates	175
Racquetball	240
Running, six miles per hour	340
Stair climber, moderate effort	300
Swimming laps, moderate effort	265
Tai chi	84
Tennis, singles	223
Tennis, doubles	125
Walking the dog	50
Walking, fast pace	160
Water aerobics	120

Weightlifting, light effort	100
Yoga, hot	240
Yoga, light effort	100
Zumba, moderate effort	245

Anaerobic Activities: What Counts?

Anaerobic activities rely on energy stored in the muscles to fuel short bursts of activity. The limiting factor of an anaerobic workout is the fatigue associated with the buildup of lactic acid in the muscles. Although you may skip fencing, hockey, and soccer, you'll definitely want to participate in other forms of anaerobic exercise.

Sprints. Sprinting enhances the body's overall metabolism rate, tones muscles, and sculpts body structure.

Isotonics. Mostly used by weightlifters, who are accustomed to lifting dumbbells/barbells on a regular basis, these exercises put muscles in continuous motion, constrained by tension through the instrument used. Isotonic exercises help in toning muscles and reducing flab. Examples include leg lunges and pull-ups.

Isometrics. Isometric exercises, which are aimed at strengthening, require muscles to exert force against hard or immovable objects (like a wall). These exercises require muscles to be held in a particular position for an extended time. Since bone joints remain stable during isometrics, muscle flexibility increases. Examples include planks, bridges, and chair pose.

Calisthenics. More commonly known as muscle-strengthening exercises, calisthenics do not involve weights or equipment. These exercises aim to improve body resistance. Examples include push-ups and squats.

Muscle Strengthening Activities: What Works?

Strength training improves muscle tone, boosts self-esteem, and helps you lose body fat. At least two days a week, all the body's major muscle groups—legs, hips, back, chest, abdomen, shoulders, and arms—need to be worked. Maximum health benefits are attained when you do muscle-strengthening exercises to the point that it's difficult to do another repetition. A repetition is one complete movement of activity, such as one push-up, or lifting a weight and returning to the starting position. One set equals eight to twelve repetitions. As you grow stronger, build from one set to two or three.

The Aerobics and Fitness Association of America recommends two to three nonconsecutive days per week of strength-building exercises. Perform eight to ten exercises for each muscle group, two to four sets, eight to twelve repetitions. Variety is important. Muscle-strengthening exercises can be performed on the same days as aerobic activity. These types of exercises can be done at home or in a gym, with weights, resistance bands, or even using your own body weight as resistance. They include:

- exercise balls
- hand weights
- heavy yard work
- lunges
- medicine balls
- resistance bands
- push-ups
- planks
- sit-ups
- yoga

If you want to achieve maximum hormonal benefits from exercise, aerobic and anaerobic, it is important to follow the dietary recommendations of our plan as part of your exercise regimen. We recommend eating a healthy snack, such as an apple or nuts, thirty minutes before exercising. In addition, be sure to drink plenty of water during the activity.

Don't forget to loosen up before and stretch well after exercising. Keeping your muscles and ligaments soft and pliable is essential to improving your overall fitness and well-being.

Get to the Core

Strengthening core muscles has been shown to reduce risk of injury, as well as improve overall health. Core-strengthening exercises are recognized by most physicians and physical therapists as important in maintaining functional posture, strengthening the body, and minimizing the risk of injury. It is important to maintain core strength in order to protect the spine from injury during such common activities as lifting groceries or carrying suitcases. Many core-strengthening exercises can easily be performed at home and should be done at least three times per week. We recommend you consult with your physician or a licensed physical therapist before beginning a core-strengthening exercise regimen.

The basis of core stabilization includes two primary steps. The first is finding a correct neutral spine. The spine has two natural curves—one at the neck and another at the lower back. If you lie on your back with both knees bent and feet flat on the surface, you should have a small space (about the size of a grape) between your back and the surface. This is your neutral spine position.

The second step is achieving a proper core contraction. To properly contract the core muscles, think about drawing your navel back toward your spine without changing the neutral spinal position. To check for proper contraction, place your index and middle fingertips just in front of the widest part of your hips (where they drop down into soft tissue). As you draw your navel in, you should feel a deep muscle contraction. It is important to maintain a natural, steady breathing pattern during this muscle contraction. Be sure that you are not holding your breath and that you are relaxed. Following is a brief description of some common exercises you can do at home to stabilize and strengthen your core.

Mat Exercises

Bridge. Lying on a flat surface, with both knees bent and feet flat on floor, find neutral spine, contract core muscles, and lift your pelvic region off the surface while maintaining neutral spine and core contraction. Hold three to five seconds and slowly lower pelvis to surface. Remember to maintain a steady breathing pattern. Work up to three sets of ten repetitions.

Partial curl-ups. On a flat surface, with both knees bent and feet flat on floor, find neutral spine, contract core muscles, and slowly slide both hands toward your knees, lifting your head and shoulders off the ground while maintaining neutral spine and core contraction. Hold three to five seconds and slowly return to resting position. Remember to maintain a steady breathing pattern. Work up to three sets of ten repetitions.

Modified push-ups. Begin on your stomach, knees bent, with both palms flat on the floor, elbows bent, and thumbs at nipple level. Find neutral spine, contract core muscles, and slowly extend both elbows until arms are straight, keeping knees on floor. Hold three to five seconds, then slowly lower body back to floor by bending elbows. Maintain neutral spine and core contraction throughout exercise. Remember to maintain steady breathing pattern. Work up to three sets of ten repetitions.

Wall squats. Standing with back toward a wall, feet shoulder-width apart, and a stability ball placed between small of back and wall surface, find neutral spine and contract core muscles. Slowly bend knees, making sure knees do not extend beyond toes. Slowly return to standing position. Maintain neutral spine and core contraction throughout exercise. Do not extend your back over top of the stability ball, and remember to maintain a steady breathing pattern. Work up to three sets of ten repetitions.

CHAPTER FOURTEEN

Stress Management

*I*t's pretty common to hear someone say, "I'm so stressed out." Our fast-paced lives are filled with responsibilities for our career, our family to care for, and bills to pay. Add to that the fact that we live in some pretty stressful times. Each year the American Psychological Association conducts a survey entitled "Stress in America." For the past few years, people have reported being worried about the future of our country, the state of healthcare, and events such as mass shootings.

Stress is so common that it is easy to take for granted as just another part of life we have to deal with. But experiencing a heightened level of stress for long periods of time can do damage to your body. Learning to recognize stress and keeping it at manageable levels can help you lead a healthier life and even stave off cognitive decline.

Stress is a feeling of emotional or physical tension. When we are constantly worried or anxious, these emotions cause wear and tear on our bodies. Some signs of stress are irritability and moodiness. We may snap at our colleagues, be short with our partners, not be as loving toward our children as we'd like to be. Stress can lead to bad sleep habits and insomnia, which in turn leads to fatigue. Other symptoms of stress include lack of energy, headaches, gastrointestinal distress, and decreased ability to focus.

Stress also affects the body in ways that aren't immediately noticeable. The body's reaction to stress is to increase production of cortisol. At high levels, cortisol is toxic to our brains. Increased cortisol can lead to high blood pressure, increased blood glucose levels, and cardiovascular disease, all of which are risk factors for cognitive decline. Cortisol also suppresses the work of the immune system, making you more likely to get sick during periods of stress.

While there's not conclusive evidence that stress directly causes Alzheimer's, the effects of stress on the body have a connection to many risk factors of Alzheimer's and cognitive decline. Hormones produced by the body during times of stress have been shown to have growth-inhibiting effects on a variety of tissues, including the brain.

When it comes to Alzheimer's disease, stress is part of a vicious cycle. Not only can stress be a risk factor in leading to development of Alzheimer's, the disease itself can cause stress. First, and maybe most obvious, a diagnosis of Alzheimer's is stressful. A decline in cognitive ability adds stress to daily activities. In addition, the loss of cognitive function that comes with Alzheimer's disease can disrupt the neural circuits that mediate the body's stress responses.

What Causes You Stress?

It is clear that managing stress levels can have many benefits, from improving your outlook on life to experiencing better health and possibly staving off cognitive decline. The first step to reducing stress and anxiety levels in your life is to understand what causes you stress. The list at the beginning of this chapter is often what comes to mind: financial worries, taking care of children or elderly parents, responsibilities at work.

In addition to the common worries of life daily life, large life events are often triggers for stress—losing a job, declaring bankruptcy, going through divorce, suffering the loss of a parent, child, or sibling, or serving in combat.

Managing Stress

Of course it's impossible to eliminate stress from your life entirely, but by becoming more aware of the stressors in your life and practicing some different stress-relief techniques, you can learn to manage stress.

Adopt healthy lifestyle habits. Getting a good night's sleep, eating healthy foods, and exercising regularly are three important ways to help lower stress levels. It's clear that we're much better able to deal with the unexpected challenges life throws at us when we're alert and well rested.

We'll cover diet in depth in part III of this book, but it's easy to see the link between a healthy diet and managing stress. The foods we eat affect how our body's systems work, and it's important not to put undue strain on those systems with highly processed and sugary foods. Cutting back on caffeine can help manage stress levels as well. Caffeine raises cortisol levels, which increases your stress levels.

Consume alcohol in moderation. Alcohol changes the levels of serotonin and other neurotransmitters in the brain, which can worsen anxiety. In some studies, mild amounts of alcohol consumption have been shown to reduce a person's risk of dementia. For men, this is no more than one to two alcoholic drinks per day. For women, no more than one drink per day is considered mild alcohol use. The bad news is that heavy drinking— more than two drinks per day—can *double* the odds of developing dementia compared to not drinking at all, and the effects are even greater in heavy drinkers who carry the ApoE4 gene. We recommend either avoiding alcohol or using it only in moderation. It is very important for people who carry the ApoE4 gene to either avoid alcohol altogether or use it only in moderation.

Express yourself. One way to figure out what life activities or events are causing you stress is through keeping a journal. The benefits of a journal are twofold, for in addition to learning what types of things cause you stress, writing about them can help you deal with your feelings. The simple act of writing these worries is a good way to let go of your anxiety and frustrations.

Journal entries can take many different forms. You might use your journal one day to write down your worries, and the next use your entry to write the things you are grateful for. Recognizing the good in your life is a positive step toward reducing stress.

Talking with someone is another good way to express your feelings. It might be a counselor, a family member, or a close friend who can allow you to talk things through and lessen your stress levels.

Manage your time wisely. The same thing your third-grade teacher said every day holds true in your adult life. Learning to say no is very important in managing stress. How many items on your calendar do you dread attending? Avoid serving on committees that don't interest you, and cut back on obligations that take up too much of your time; instead spend your time on the activities and events you truly enjoy.

Managing your time includes learning how to set boundaries when it comes to work. As much as possible, put the cell phone away and save emails and texts for the hours when you're at work, rather than during your personal time.

Use your vacation days. Taking time off to relax and unwind is important, and too many of us aren't taking advantage of it as often as we should. According to the US Travel Association, more than half of Americans have unused vacations days at the end of the year. Part of that comes from the feeling of "not having time to take time off," but studies show vacations actually improve productivity.

Practice relaxation techniques. Something as simple as taking a deep breath can help lower your anxiety levels. When you breathe deeply, your body sends a message to your brain to calm down and relax, which in turn helps decrease the symptoms of stress: increased heart rate, rapid breathing, and high blood pressure. Belly breathing is one type of deep breathing exercises to try. First, sit or lie in a comfortable position, placing one hand on your belly just below your ribs and your other hand on your chest. Take a deep breath in through your nose and let your belly push your hand out. Your chest should not move. Then breathe out through your lips as if you are whistling. Use the hand on your belly to help push all the air out.

Meditation is another practice that can reduce stress. Meditation isn't about changing who you are, but about training yourself to achieve an emotionally calm and stable state. The practice of relaxation and breathing techniques evolved thousands of years ago as a means to explore the inner being and expand self-awareness. Meditation can be practiced by anyone, anywhere.

Scientific studies have proven that meditation has significant effects on the brain. Meditation slows down brain activity, significantly reducing stress, improving circulation, reducing anxiety, lowering heart rate, decreasing chronic pain, and, ultimately, reducing signs of aging. Just twenty minutes of meditation per day can cut the progression rate of cognitive impairment in half. In his book *Tools of Titans: The Tactics, Routines, and Habits of Billionaires, Icons, and World-Class Performers*, author Tim Ferriss revealed that more than 80 percent of his interviewees had some form of daily mindfulness or meditation practice.[21]

There are different techniques used for meditation, including practicing mindfulness, or focusing the mind on a particular object. Just say "Om."

A good way to learn about and start practicing meditation is through an app on your smartphone or tablet. Several different apps, such as Headspace, Calm, and Simple Habit, provide good introductions to the practices of meditation and guided meditation. There are also many excellent podcasts that can help with your practice. Mindfulness-based stress reduction (MBSR), developed by Professor Jon Kabat-Zinn, is an eight-week evidence-based program that trains people to cultivate awareness.

Take up yoga. Combining exercise, controlled breathing, and meditation, the practice of yoga goes a long way toward helping alleviate stress. Studies have found that practicing yoga helps modulate the body's stress response, which in turn reduces the heart rate and lowers blood pressure. There are many different ways to get involved with yoga, from signing up for a class at a local gym to following a YouTube video. One of the nice things about yoga is that practicing just a few poses for a few minutes a day can be beneficial.

Practice tai chi. Tai chi has also been proven to help with stress. It's a low-impact, traditional Chinese form of exercise that is accessible for most seniors. It promotes deep breathing, reduces blood pressure, releases endorphins, enhances mental capacity and concentration, and many other benefits. The Chinese practice this in public parks and it's now sweeping across America.

Take time to find a few ways to manage stress that can be easily incorporated into your daily routine. You don't have to do everything on this list. Find the practices you enjoy, and you'll be more apt to make them part of your daily routine.

CHAPTER FIFTEEN

Brain Stimulation

*T*he slogan "use it or lose it" is bandied about quite regularly with trainers and in gyms. If you've ever embarked on a program to train for and run a 5K, you are familiar with the aptness of this saying. Say, for example, you work up to being able to run three and a half miles, participate in a few races, and then slack off on your training once you don't have any races on the schedule. When you go back to run again a few months later, you find it's just as hard to run that first mile as it was when you started. Your body works up its muscle strength and endurance levels, and can lose it when not working out regularly.

The same is true for your brain. Learning new things and keeping your mind active are as important to maintaining good cognitive abilities throughout your life as a healthy diet, regular exercise, good sleep, and stress management.

For years, researchers have found that people with high levels of education and intellectually stimulating careers have lower risk of developing dementia. People who spend more time engaging their minds over their lifetime (in school, in their careers, or just in self-disciplined learning like reading books or taking classes for fun) have been shown to develop more robust networks of nerve cells and connections within the brain. This, in turn, means the brain is better equipped to handle cell damage that may lead to dementia and Alzheimer's disease.

Not only can exercising the brain help delay the onset of symptoms of dementia or Alzheimer's, it might help slow the decline in people diagnosed with the disease. Studies have shown that reasoning exercises—things like crossword puzzles, Sudoku, games like Scrabble, and word-finding games—can improve mental function in people with some cognitive decline.

It's easy to equate brain function with activities like crosswords and reading, but social stimulation is also a vital part of brain stimulation and health. Research at the Rush University Medical Center in Chicago found that having close friends and staying in contact with family members helps protect the brain against the effects of Alzheimer's.

While maintaining relationships with friends and family can have a protective effect on the brain, the lack of relationships can have the opposite effect. Researchers in Spain studied a compilation of studies from the United States and Europe and found that loneliness was associated with a 26 percent increased risk of dementia. One of the studies found a 105 percent increased risk of mild cognitive impairment linked to loneliness.

It's Never Too Late to Learn Something New

One of the important steps in keeping your brain active is to make cognitive activities a part of your daily routine, just like getting regular physical exercise. Becoming a couch potato after retirement isn't just bad for your blood pressure; it's bad for your brain as well. One way to find new cognitive activities and keep to a regular schedule is through an app such as Lumosity, Elevate, or BrainHQ. These apps have scientifically developed games that help improve cognition through reading and math activities. They even track your progress, so you can see the results for yourself.

You don't have to reach for your smartphone or tablet to complete some brain exercises each day. Word and number puzzles and other types of brain puzzles serve the same effect. Get out your paper and pencil, and in this case keep away from your screens so you're not tempted to let Google help you out when you're stumped.

There are many other ways to exercise your brain even when you're no longer a student with homework every day.

Learn a new language. It might be a little more challenging for older people to learn a language than it is for children, but that doesn't mean it can't be done. Sign up for a class or try an app like Duolingo or Babbel to help get you on your way to becoming multilingual. Practice your new skills by reading a newspaper from the country where your language of choice is spoken, or plan a trip to get firsthand experience conversing with others.

Learn a new skill. Taking on a new challenge such as learning electrical wiring, furniture upholstery, or winemaking can keep your brain working as well. Look for courses at a local community college that might interest you. You may just find yourself sprucing up your own home or completing a project you otherwise would have had to pay someone else to do.

Make the most of your hobbies. Knitting, cross-stitch, quilting, painting, woodworking, gardening, and cooking are just a few enjoyable ways to pass the time and utilize brain cells at the same time. Retired or not, it's important to find time in your life to spend on the hobbies you enjoy. If you don't happen to have a hobby, it's a great time to learn something new.

Building Your Social Network

Social networks aren't just for Mark Zuckerberg. Maintaining relationships with friends and family might take some effort on your part, but the benefits are well worth the effort.

Get out around people. Many of us already have social networks built in to our daily lives. Church, work, and clubs are all places we're around other people and get a chance to make small talk and catch up on news, events, movies, or books. But it doesn't help much if you just attend a meeting or sit in the pew and don't interact with others. If you're a member of a church, join a small group Bible study or a Sunday school class for more personal interaction. If you like to read, find a book club at your local library or bookstore. There are also many different community service organizations such as

Lions, Rotary, and Civitan clubs that not only do good works in the community but have meetings where you can socialize with others on a regular basis.

Set up a regular time to meet with friends. Who hasn't been guilty of telling your friends you need to get together, but not following through? The best way to nurture those relationships is to set a regular date. This can be of particular importance once you enter retirement. I know of one example of a church not far from my home city of Charlotte where the preacher made a pot of coffee every day at ten o'clock and made it known that he would welcome company. Within a few weeks, a group of men were gathering for an hour or so of drinking coffee and talking after the morning chores were done. (The group wasn't limited to men; it just so happened that's who showed up. Maybe their wives already had regular social outlets.) The great thing about this example is the dependability of the gathering. The same can be done anywhere. Make a commitment to a friend to meet for lunch once a week, or set up a time with your daughter for a phone or video call when you know she's not busy with work. Having a plan not only encourages you to socialize, it gives you something to look forward to.

Make new friends. If there's one thing in life that's constant, it's change. Sometimes the people you're close to become unavailable for social time, for various reasons. In this case, it's helpful to have a few places where you can make new friendships and keep your network large and healthy. The clubs and activities listed above are good avenues to meet new people, as are senior centers and exercise classes.

Getting the Best of Both Worlds

Brain stimulation comes in the form of both mental activities and social engagement, but the two are so interconnected that many of the ideas here can't clearly be divided out as serving just one function or the other. For example, learning a new activity or hobby can be educational, but also social if you're part of a class or take a trip with a group of fellow travelers. Joining a book club is a good way to make friends, and you get the added benefit of reading a new book and having a fruitful discussion. A couple of other ideas for keeping your brain healthy that encompass both the mental and the social aspect are:

Card games. Other than solitaire, it's impossible to play a card game alone. Keep that brain sharp with a game of bridge or gin rummy, and make it a date by setting up a regular game night or joining a group of competitors.

Volunteering opportunities. Tutoring local school kids in math, science, or reading is a good way to keep up on the latest trends and have some interesting conversations along the way. Schools aren't the only places looking for volunteers; there's plenty of need at animal shelters, hospitals, libraries, and food banks . . . the list goes on!

It really doesn't matter what type of activity you do. The important thing is to keep your brain working. Find something that interests you and make it a part of your routine. When you can bring along a friend or family member to enjoy it with you, you benefit even more. Find your passion and get enthusiastic about your overall health and well-being.

CHAPTER SIXTEEN

Top 20 List for Improving Your Mind and Living a Healthier Life

Top 20 things you can do to prevent Alzheimer's disease.

1. **Get Moving.** Daily exercise is essential for a healthy body and a healthy brain!

2. **Sleep well.** Make sure you are getting the sleep you need each night. Most of us need between seven and eight hours of quality sleep each night.

3. **Break a bad habit.** If you smoke . . . stop! When it comes to healthy living, nothing you do matters more than breaking your nicotine habit.

4. **Play mind games.** Stimulate your mind. A growing amount of research reveals the importance of limiting your screen time and stimulating your mind through reading, education, and intellectual activities.

5. **Reduce stress.** Chronic stress creates overproduction of hormones like cortisol, which can cause damage to cells in the memory center of the brain. Successful stress management includes meditation, yoga, tai chi, and many other techniques that can promote relaxation and help you deal more effectively with stressful situations.

6. **Keep your blood pressure down**. Uncontrolled blood pressure can more than quintuple your risk of dementia. Follow your doctor's advice and work to get your blood pressure under 120/80.

7. **Know your numbers.** Control your cholesterol and your blood-sugar levels. Work with your healthcare team to keep your cholesterol and glucose levels within normal limits.

8. **Lose weight.** Obesity promotes inflammation, shrinks your brain, and sets the stage for dementia.

9. **Have your hearing checked.** Decreased hearing can significantly increase the risk of Alzheimer's disease.

10. **Fight inflammation.** Consider having your CRP levels checked, and ask your doctor what you can do to reduce the levels of inflammation in your system.

11. **Hydrate.** Start your day with a large glass of purified water. Drinking five to six glasses of pure water each day is the best way to flush the body and the brain of toxins and waste, and rehydrate every cell in your body.

12. **Eat real food that nourishes your body and work to avoid processed foods.**

13. **Get most of your vitamins and minerals from the foods you eat.** Exceptions that may require supplements are omega-3 fatty acids, vitamin D, turmeric, and some B vitamins.

14. **Decrease your intake of animal protein, including dairy, and limit red meat to once a week.**

15. **Eat a rainbow of colorful foods every day.** Feast on fresh fruits and vegetables.

16. **Eat or drink something fermented each day.**

17. **Skip the sugar.** Too much glucose in the diet has been linked to diabetes, cardiovascular disease, stroke, and Alzheimer's disease.

18. **Limit alcohol intake.** More than one to two drinks per day can be toxic to your brain and your overall health.

19. **Avoid environmental toxins and activity that could lead to concussions.**

20. **Keep mentally active.** Learn something new. Rekindle old friendships.

Bonus Tip

Be enthusiastic—no other human characteristic contributes so much to happiness and healthy living.

PART III

Healthy Eating for a Sharper Mind

CHAPTER SEVENTEEN

Eat as We Were Designed

Cheryl's Story

I am a registered pharmacist and a cancer survivor, and I am certified in plant-based nutrition. I started this journey many years ago when I decided to go to pharmacy school. I ended up working in all areas of pharmacy, first as a pharmaceutical sales representative, then as a hospital pharmacist in two different teaching hospitals, and finally in a retail pharmacy setting. After my cancer diagnosis, I put my science background to work, researching how I could properly nourish my body to fight further disease and stay as healthy as possible. I went to seminars, conferences, and continuing-education classes; got certified in plant-based nutrition; and read everything I could find on nourishing our bodies well.

After much research, I realized there was actually a pharmacy in my kitchen that I could use every day. I discovered that every bite you take is an opportunity to help your body fight disease. I also discovered the shocking truth that people are fed by the food industry, which pays no attention to health, and are treated by the health industry, which pays no attention to food. The only good news is that *you* have control over how you nourish and take care of your body, and it does indeed make a tremendous difference in your health. I started Pharmacy In Your Kitchen and began to teach others how to do what I had learned to do. Now I'm sharing that knowledge with you.

—Cheryl Hoover, RPh

The Pharmacy In Your Kitchen Philosophy

I believe we were carefully and perfectly designed. As such, our bodies were made to fight disease and stay healthy. If you have ever watched a wound heal over the course of several days or had a broken bone or a damaged nerve that healed over time, you have seen this beautiful design in action. If we are properly nourished, our bodies can do what they were designed to do: stay healthy. When we are not nourished well, our bodies become stressed and distracted, and they cannot do this very important job. When we deprive our bodies of the raw materials they need to function properly, we are creating an environment of chronic inflammation and imbalances that, over time, manifests in chronic disease progression. That's when we become sick.

Our brains were designed to make new neural connections, new brain cells, and to positively adapt in response to our environment by a process called neuroplasticity. Brain-derived neurotrophic factor (BDNF) is a protein that promotes neuroplasticity. Having enough BDNF around can protect our brains from neurodegenerative diseases and our hearts from heart disease. The food you eat plays a pivotal role in whether this neuroplasticity can happen. Eliminating sugar, processed foods, and high-fructose corn syrup from your diet, and replacing them with things like oily fish, olive oil, curry, turmeric, red grapes, and blueberries, will feed your brain properly to allow this process to occur.

Another process that we need to pay attention to regarding brain health is inflammation. The root of many major illnesses in this country is chronic inflammation. The primary source of inflammation in a typical standard American diet is animal protein. In addition to directly causing inflammation, when we fill our plate with animal protein, it does not allow room on the plate or in our belly for the number and diversity of plants we should be eating.

Diets high in polyphenols, i.e., colorful fruits and vegetables, are shown to reduce oxidative stress and inflammation. Simply said, eat a rainbow of colorful plants, which is where all the nutrients your brain and body need can be found. Proper nourishment fuels your body with foods that do not cause inflammation or stress, but instead offer nutrients your body needs and was designed to use.

Real food was put here on earth to nourish our bodies, while food-like substances are made in factories and are preserved and processed. The food industry has changed our food expectations and even our taste buds, but we still choose what to eat. The standard American diet (SAD) is lacking in whole foods, fiber, and phytonutrients, marked by excessive meat consumption, and laden with refined sugar and alternative sweeteners, processed and refined foods, synthetic chemicals, neurotoxic food dyes, and oxidized vegetable oils.

We recommend decreasing the amount of animal protein you eat and avoiding manmade foods. Manmade foods are highly processed foods and chemicals that offer little nutritional value and are hardly recognized by our bodies as fuel. These products lack the nutrients we need and leave us consuming empty calories that cause our bodies stress.

Decrease Animal Protein

What is an animal protein, and why do we typically eat so much of it? Animal protein includes meat, eggs, cheese, milk, ice cream, yogurt, and butter. If you go back just two or three generations in Americans, you will find that meat and animal products were not an every-meal occurrence. People raised their own food and ate mostly fresh, seasonal fruits and vegetables. When they did eat animal protein, they knew where it came from and how it was raised. Beans, rice, and other grains were what typically complemented the fruits and vegetables on the plate. We were not an affluent country, so we ate more like paupers, not kings. When we became a wealthier nation, we ultimately became a sicker nation. Turns out eating like kings is actually very harmful to our health.

If you choose to eat animal protein, think of it more as a "condiment" on your plate rather than the main attraction. It is also important, if you choose to eat meat, that the animal was fed its natural diet, not a cheaper alternative, and was not pumped with antibiotics. Cows should be grass-fed instead of grain-fed, pasture-raised instead of factory-farmed.

People worry that they won't get enough protein if they don't eat a lot of meat. Turns out we don't need as much protein as the meat and dairy industries would like you to believe. You can get all the protein you need from a whole-food plant-based diet rich in seeds, nuts, beans, legumes, fruits, and vegetables. If you eat real food rich in fiber and nutrients and are not losing weight, chances are you are getting enough protein in your diet.

Fish

If you're going to eat animal protein, fish can be a better choice than land-based animals. Stay away from eating really big fish, like tuna or swordfish. Small fish are less likely than bigger fish to have accumulated toxins in them. This is a natural result of the aquatic food chain: the bigger the fish, the more likely they are to have eaten other fish that have accumulated toxins. Medium-sized fish like flounder and salmon are better choices, and smaller fish like sardines and anchovies are healthy choices. While the "wild-caught" label may seem virtuous, farm-raised fish also have the potential to be healthy, if they are fed their natural diet, live in a clean environment, and are not pumped with antibiotics. However, some farm-raised fish are fed corn and soy that has been genetically modified. These seeds, called genetically modified organisms (GMOs), are obviously not a part of their natural diet. Wild salmon flesh is pink due to their natural diet, which is rich in carotenoids. The feed of farm-raised salmon has added pigmenting compounds to produce pink flesh; otherwise it would be gray.

Eggs

As an animal protein, eggs should be eaten sparingly, and the quality of the egg is important too. The labels "free-range" and "natural" mean nothing. Look for "organic," which means the birds were fed their natural diet and no antibiotics were used. Ideally, get to know your farmer, and try to buy from someone who raises the birds in as close to their natural environment as possible. A happy chicken lays a healthy egg.

Eat Real Food

Today, we are a nation that craves food that didn't even exist a few generations ago, like fast food. If you look at what is offered in the center aisles of the grocery store, you will see that most of that food is manmade and full of preservatives. Just a few years ago, people didn't even know what a probiotic was; now many people take one as a supplement because the standard American diet is so bad for our gut health. And as it turns out, if your gut is unhealthy, then even if you eat well, your body will not fully be able to utilize the food to properly nourish your body.

Your food *should* expire. If it doesn't, you shouldn't eat it. Eat things that were grown in the ground, things that will spoil if not refrigerated, things that have a limited shelf life or will spoil over time. To take this one step further, you might say, "If God didn't make it, try not to eat it." Put whole, real food in your body and avoid artificial ingredients, preservatives, and manmade foods.

Read labels and compare products based on their ingredients. Shop the perimeter of the grocery store—the produce and refrigerated sections—and eat seasonally. Fortunately, more and more people are becoming educated about their food, which makes it easier to make good decisions about your food choices. Just make the best decisions you can with the options you have in front of you.

Eat Organic When Possible

Conventionally farmed fruits and vegetables are often grown in mineral-deficient soil. They look pretty but are nutrient poor. In addition to this, they're sprayed with pesticides that our bodies were not designed to ingest. Even if you can't get everything organic, try to at least buy the "dirty dozen" organic. Every year the Environmental Working Group publishes an updated list with the top twelve fruits and vegetables that you should buy organic in order to avoid ingesting pesticides and chemicals. Again, do the best you can with the choices you have in front of you.

Avoid GMOs

GMOs are genetically modified organisms, designed in a laboratory to be resistant to pesticides and herbicides so farmers can spray their fields to control insects and weeds. These man-made GMO grains are then sprayed with more chemicals right before harvest to speed up the dehydration process. They are then turned into food products laden with chemicals that you unknowingly eat. Most of the corn, soy, and canola oil in the United States is GMO, unless it specifically says it is non-GMO or organic. Genetically modified foods are not what your body was designed to eat in the first place, but the chemicals applied not only during the growth process but specifically right before harvest make these products something to be avoided at all costs.

Eat Natural Fats

Your body needs fat to flourish, but only good fats. Good fats are found in whole foods like avocados, nuts, seeds, fatty fish, and olive oil. When you eat an olive, you can't help but believe it was easy to make oil from it; extra-virgin olive oil is simply what drains out of crushed olives, without any chemicals or refining. But think about how much processing, refining, and manipulating it takes to make oil from corn! It's common sense: eat as true to the origin of your foods' roots as possible.

Eat the Rainbow

Another thing I say all the time is, "Eat the rainbow every day, but not the same rainbow every day." Vegetables and fruits in a wide range of colors should make up most of your diet. Intense color indicates powerful phytonutrients—plant substances that are beneficial to our health—and getting a variety of these every day is very important to your overall best health. However, eating well but eating the same thing every day is not ideal. Fruits and vegetables fall into five different color categories: green, orange/yellow, red, blue/purple, and white/brown. Each fruit and vegetable color group carries its own unique disease-fighting nutrients. These phytonutrients are responsible for the vibrant colors and healthy properties of the foods that should make up at least 75 percent of your daily food intake.

Eat Seasonally and Locally When Possible

Your body was designed to eat many different foods throughout the year. It is not by chance that different foods grow in different seasons in different climates. If we were supposed to eat an apple every day, they would be available on the trees every-where, every day. They are not. People who live in a warm climate most of the year have different nutritional needs from those who live in a colder climate that has less sunlight throughout the year. Our world food-supply system has caused us to forget what grows in what season and where it grows, because we can get anything delivered to our grocery stores any time of year. Eating seasonally also encourages you to eat locally, which decreases the amount of time your food travels to you. Since fruits and vegetables begin to lose nutrition as soon as they are picked, local produce is delivered to you with much higher nutritional value than produce that's been shipped from another part of the world.

Avoid Sugar and Artificial Sweeteners

I suggest avoiding sugar unless it is in its natural form. Anything processed or manmade is unhealthy for your gut and overall health. The natural sugar in whole fruits and vegetables is designed to be eaten with the fiber in the whole food. Our bodies are meant to metabolize sugar in this way, not as tablespoonfuls of white sugar that have been bleached and processed. We know that sugar has been linked to an increased risk of heart disease, cancer, diabetes, and Alzheimer's. If you want to sweeten your food, try to use maple syrup, honey, and dates. Also, be careful with fruit juices; again, our bodies are meant to process whole fruits, not to drink the juice of several fruits in a large glass.

Don't Be Afraid of Good Carbohydrates

Try to avoid wheat, especially if it was grown in the United States. Much of the wheat in this country has been stripped of its whole grain, processed, bleached, and modified to contain more gluten than original wheat. This results in more and more people suffering from gluten sensitivities and gluten intolerance. Instead, explore alternatives like farro, spelt, barley, oats, and quinoa. These ancient grains have been minimally changed by selective breeding, as opposed to corn, white rice, and most wheat. They are higher in fiber and overall a better choice than anything white or wheat. Other good carbohydrates to incorporate into your diet regularly are fruits and vegetables. Choose whole, real food, and you can eat carbohydrates and nourish your body.

Fermented Foods and Gut Health

The pharmacist in me has noticed that many people today take supplemental fiber and probiotics. The general public didn't even know what a probiotic was fifteen years ago, but our gut health has gotten so bad that we need to take a supplement to try to add in good bacteria for proper gut balance. And fiber is the number one thing missing in the American diet. Why? Because we have replaced real, whole foods with high-sugar, high-fat foods stripped of fiber and nutrition, and it's destroying the ideal balance of good and bad bacteria in our intestinal system. If your intestinal system (your gut), is not healthy, you begin to suffer from all sorts of diseases, including colitis, diverticulitis, and leaky gut syndrome. When these things start to happen, it is very hard for your body to get the proper nourishment it needs to fight other diseases.

In addition to a whole-food diet, you should also aim to eat or drink something fermented every day. Some common fermented foods are sauerkraut (fermented cabbage), miso (fermented soybean paste), kombucha (fermented tea), tempeh (fermented soybeans), kimchi (fermented seasoned vegetables), and kefir (fermented milk). They have live bacteria in them and can restore your gut health to a place of good balance where it can absorb the nutrients needed to fuel your body well.

Be a Nutritarian

Becoming a vegan or vegetarian does not automatically mean you are eating healthy. A nutritarian looks for the best nutritional value in what they choose to eat. Eat real foods full of natural fiber and nutrients, and avoid anything manmade and void of nutrition. Stay away from chemicals and preservatives. Read food labels. If you can't pronounce it and it doesn't grow in nature, try not to eat it.

A Daily Plan for Your Success

Breakfast

We suggest you fill your first meal of the day with whatever you find hardest to fit into your diet. If you're not sure you're eating enough fruit, start your day off with it to ensure that you're eating plenty of it. If you're in a hurry or traveling, you might just have berries and nuts for breakfast. Some easy breakfast suggestions if you have more time: oatmeal with fresh berries, an ancient-grain bread with almond butter and fresh peaches, or avocado and tomatoes on your morning toast. Eat anything you like that is full of nutrients and void of sugar, empty calories, and fake ingredients. Breakfast can even be leftovers from last night's meal—it doesn't have to be what we think of as traditional breakfast food. Typical American breakfast choices are high in sugar and low in nutrients: waffles with syrup, doughnuts, and sugary cereals. These are not what we should be nourishing our body with.

Contrary to popular belief, breakfast is not always the most important meal of the day. Occasionally, you might try intermittent fasting by avoiding eating after dinner until lunchtime the next day. This temporary fasting allows your body to naturally repair itself as it was designed to do, instead of constantly digesting and metabolizing foods.

Lunch

Lunch is a time to eat a rainbow of vegetables in a salad, or have a broth-based soup or leftovers from a previous healthy meal. Limit your land animal protein here, or even better, eliminate it totally at this point in your day. Try beans, lentils, tofu, or fish in place of traditional chicken or beef. You will miss the animal protein less than you think, and you will be making room on your plate for the foods that have the nutrients your body needs.

Soup for lunch is a wonderful way to eat well. It is the perfect way to use healthy ingredients in appropriate proportions. Healthy soups start with a broth and have lots of vegetables, and usually have only a small amount of animal protein, if any. They are typically filling, nutritious, and often seasonal as well.

Dinner

At dinner, try to fill your plate with whatever you have missed during the day. Your dinner should be mostly veggies; I suggest at least two or three different varieties of vegetable. They should be the majority of your meal, and you should try to include as many different colors of the rainbow as possible. If you do choose to have an animal protein for dinner, try to think of it as an enhancement to the vegetables instead of the star of the show. Fill your plate with foods that have the nutrients your body needs to heal and stay healthy.

Snacks

Snack if you're hungry, but not because you're bored. Actually, if you think you're hungry and it's not a time when you normally eat, try drinking water or kombucha. Studies have shown that often we confuse hunger for thirst. If you are indeed hungry, this is another opportunity to fuel your body with food that will nourish it instead of with empty calories. Easy snacks are veggies with hummus, fresh fruit, and nuts. Avoid eating peanuts on a regular basis. They are inflammatory and not actually a nut. All the tree nuts are very good for you and do not cause inflammation. You can eat fresh fruit or dried, but be careful of added sugars in some dried fruits. Again, read the labels and try not to eat anything that you can't pronounce or that is not a natural ingredient. Even snacks are important decisions and an opportunity to choose well.

Learning to eat in ways that support your body's best functioning is a journey. As you change your habits, your cravings will change too. Work toward progress, not perfection.

CHAPTER EIGHTEEN

Ingredients

*T*here is a culinary pharmacy in your kitchen just waiting for you to tap in to it to nourish your body with the nutrients it needs to fight disease and be healthy. Although this list is not by any means complete, it does highlight the ingredients used in the recipes that follow.

Almonds. We have known for years that almonds are heart healthy and a wonderful source of protein, fiber, and healthy fat. Anything that is good for your heart is equally good for your brain health. Almonds decrease oxidative stress and inflammation, they are considered one of the best nutritional sources of vitamin E, and they are high in magnesium and manganese. Adding almonds into your diet is a wonderful way to improve your diet and overall health.

Apricots. The beautiful orange color of this fruit provides beta-carotene, an antioxidant that helps prevent cognitive decline and dementia. Apricots also are rich in iron, and vitamins A and C, all of which are important in maintaining proper brain function.

Apples. This wonderful fruit comes in many colors and varieties. The fiber and vitamin C in apples is indisputably beneficial for cognitive function and cardiovascular and gut health.

Arugula. This peppery salad green is a member of the cruciferous family (which includes broccoli, cabbage, cauliflower, and kale, among others). Arugula is a nutrient-dense green that is high in fiber and phytonutrients. It works as an antioxidant and provides folate and essential minerals for your brain. In addition, cruciferous vegetables are important cancer-fighting tools and in general very good foods to incorporate into your diet.

Asparagus. This spring vegetable provides thiamine and riboflavin, as well as cancer-fighting, anti-inflammatory, and antioxidant benefits. All of these are good for the brain and cardiovascular system, which are tied together since improved cardiovascular health facilitates brain functioning. One cup of asparagus provides 3 grams of plant protein and is a great example of how to meet your protein needs with plants.

Avocados. The avocado has become very popular in recent years because of its healthy monounsaturated fats, which decrease inflammation and lower your risk of cardiac disease and cancer. We now know that anything healthy for your heart is equally healthy for your brain and results in better cognitive functioning, and the avocado is no exception.

Basil. This herb is rich in flavonoids that help with cognitive functioning. It also is rich in magnesium, which has been shown to improve memory and cognitive ability. As a side benefit, it promotes sleep, key to good brain health and functioning. Basil also helps protect from free-radical cell damage and keeps our cells healthy.

Beets. Beets are high in nitrites (not to be confused with nitrates), which increase blood flow to the brain. They also provide folate, vitamin B9, and carotenoids, all of which are essential to boosting brain functioning. As a side benefit, they are high in fiber, which is lacking in our typical American diet and needed for good gut health. A cup of beets provides 3 grams of fiber, 12 percent of the recommended daily allowance.

Beans. Using a variety of beans in your diet allows you to reduce the amount of animal protein you consume. Beans are anti-inflammatory (as opposed to animal protein, which causes inflammation). Beans are high in fiber, which is necessary for a healthy gut and microbiome, and decreases inflammation. Any time you can reduce the inflammation in your body you will feel the health benefits, and beans are a delicious way to do so.

Brussels sprouts. The cruciferous vegetables are among the healthiest of food choices, and Brussels sprouts are a wonderful example of this. They are high in vitamins K and C, both of which increase cognitive function and promote brain health. They are also cancer-fighting, high in fiber, and overall an excellent food to add to your diet.

Butternut squash. Typically the winter squashes are more nutritious than others, and butternut is no exception. It is rich in vitamins A and C, which help with cell growth and reduction of free radicals. The bright-orange color of this squash provides carotenoids that are essential for the body to make active forms of vitamin A. Finally, this squash is high in vitamin E, an antioxidant that decreases free radical damage.

Cabbage. A powerhouse vegetable in the cruciferous family, cabbage decreases inflammation and provides vitamins K and C, as well as plenty of soluble plant fiber. In addition, it comes in colors of purple, green, and white, all offering slightly different beneficial phytochemicals, so take advantage of all your options. Fermented cabbage, in the form of sauerkraut or kimchi, is a wonderful way to add the gut-health benefits of fermented foods to your diet.

Carrots. Carrots are a very heart-healthy vegetable, and again, what's good for your heart is equally good for your brain. This root vegetable provides many healthy nutrients that your body needs to protect its cells and function properly, in particular vitamins K and A, which help decrease oxidative stress.

Cashews. These nuts are an excellent source of vitamins, minerals, and antioxidants. Specifically, they provide high levels of zinc, thiamine, magnesium, and vitamin E, all of which are essential for more mental energy and better cognition. They also provide plant-based protein as well as monounsaturated fat, and are delicious as a stand-alone snack or in many recipes.

Cauliflower. Another stellar member of the cruciferous family, cauliflower provides antioxidants, folate, and vitamins K and C. This vegetable boosts overall brain functioning, memory, and mood, and is a powerful cancer-fighter as well.

Cherries. This delicious stone fruit provides a natural source of melatonin and is high in vitamin C, both of which promote proper brain functioning. The antioxidants in this fruit allow for proper cell repair and maintenance, which are essential for your overall health and cancer prevention. If you choose dried cherries, be sure to check the label for added sugar.

Chia seeds. These powerful little seeds are rich in omega-3 fatty acids, iron, fiber, and antioxidants. In general, seeds and nuts are a wonderful thing to add to your diet when you can sneak them in. These seeds are worth seeking out and adding to some of your favorite recipes. They can even serve as an egg replacement in some baked goods.

Chickpeas (also called garbanzo beans). This is a delicious bean that I tend to use often due to its versatility and nutritional attributes. Chickpeas have powerful antioxidants, folate, and magnesium—all essential for proper cell functioning and good brain health. They are high in fiber and protein, and are an easy bean to digest. They are a great addition to salads, wonderful as a hummus, and delicious roasted or in soups.

Chili (dried ground). This powerful spice uses capsaicin to fire up your brain and improve cognitive functioning. It is also rich in vitamin A, which is necessary for proper cell repair and a valuable antioxidant.

Cinnamon. This ancient spice provides anti-inflammatory benefits, aids in digestion and appetite, and has a neurotropic effect on brain cells, allowing the brain to generate new neurons and keep the old ones healthy. This spice is easy to add to a smoothie or to your coffee before it is brewed, and can be used in both sweet and savory recipes.

Coriander. These seeds are rich in vitamin K, which improves cognitive function and has been linked to improved memory. Cilantro and coriander come from the same plant but have a very different taste; cilantro is the plant (leaves and stems), and coriander are the seeds from the plant. People who dislike cilantro may still enjoy ground coriander seeds.

Corn. Corn is actually the seed of a plant in the grass family. It comes in a variety of colors and is rich in antioxidants, magnesium, fiber, vitamin C and B vitamins, all of which are important to good brain health and nourishment. There is a difference, however, between whole corn and corn that has been processed into oil. Whole corn is in its natural state, while corn oil has been refined and processed in order to turn it into oil. Don't add corn oil into your diet, but instead use corn in its natural state or ground, as in grits.

Cranberries. Cranberries are a member of the heather family and are related to blueberries and lingonberries. They boast several vitamins and minerals, including manganese, copper, and vitamins C, E, and K. Though they offer many nutritional benefits, use dried cranberries in moderation because they usually come presweetened.

Cumin. Cumin is the second-most popular spice in the world after black pepper. Aside from cooking, cumin has been used medicinally in many parts of the world for years. The seeds are usually ground into a powder and are a typical ingredient in curry spice blends. Cumin provides calcium, magnesium, and brain-boosting iron, and may improve cognitive function, appetite, and digestion.

Curry. Curry is a combination of spices, usually including ground turmeric, cumin, coriander, ginger, and dried chilies. If you are lucky enough to like this wonderfully powerful spice combination, use it often and enjoy the nutritional benefits. In addition to the attributes of cumin, chilies, and coriander above, the anti-inflammatory effects of turmeric and ginger make this spice combination a nutritional powerhouse.

Edamame. Soybeans that are green and still in their pod are called edamame. They are a wonderful source of plant protein, are available frozen, and do not require presoaking like other beans. They are rich in folate, manganese, and vitamin K, and are a wonderful anti-inflammatory to add to your diet.

Eggs. Eggs are loaded with nutrients that improve mental focus and function. One of these is choline, which is used to build cell membranes, and has a role in producing signaling molecules in the brain. Using pasture-raised, organic eggs from chickens that are fed their natural diet is the best option if you choose to eat eggs.

Farro. Farro is a very nutritious ancient grain; however, it does contain gluten. Ancient grains are generally higher in fiber and more nutritious than grains that have been processed or changed over the years. Farro is an excellent source of protein, magnesium, zinc, and B vitamins. Overall, this is an excellent grain choice for optimal health and wellness.

Garlic. Considered an herb, garlic is closely related to onions and has for years been revered for its medicinal properties; it was prescribed by the ancient Greek physician Hippocrates two thousand years ago. Garlic promotes good cardiovascular health, is strongly associated with better brain function, and has cancer-fighting properties. Garlic contains antioxidants that support the body's protective mechanisms against oxidative stress. Garlic should be incorporated into your diet daily as it is a stellar ingredient for your best overall health.

Ginger. Ginger has a very long history of use in various forms of medicine. It has been used to help digestion, reduce nausea, and help fight the common cold. It is an antioxidant powerhouse shown to boost memory skills and the ability to focus.

Grapefruit. When grapefruit is in season, take advantage of all this citrus fruit has to offer. It is rich in fiber, vitamins A and C, and flavanones, which have anti-inflammatory properties. They are a healthy choice for the cardiovascular system, the brain, and overall good health.

Halibut. Halibut is a good source of a variety of micronutrients that contribute to good health. This fish provides vitamins D and A, omega-3 fatty acids, niacin, and magnesium. In addition, the selenium content in halibut helps reduce oxidative stress and inflammation. This results in better neuronal and overall health.

Hemp seeds. Technically a nut, hemp seeds are very nutritious. They have a mild, nutty flavor and are often referred to as hemp hearts. Hemp seeds are rich in healthy fats, protein, and minerals such as phosphorus, potassium, sodium, magnesium, sulfur, calcium, iron, and zinc. They are considered a complete protein source, which means that they provide all the essential amino acids your body needs. They are high in fiber, easy to digest, and a wonderful addition to your diet.

Kale. Often called a "super green," kale is loaded with all sorts of beneficial compounds with medicinal properties. This leafy cruciferous vegetable is one of the most nutrient-dense foods you can add to your diet. Many important minerals are found in kale, some of which are lacking in the modern diet, including calcium, potassium, and magnesium. Kale is high in vitamins C and K, as well as beta-carotene, an antioxidant that the body converts to vitamin A. Some people find kale a bit hard to chew and digest if eaten raw. If I serve kale raw, I chop the leaves and massage them with some lemon juice, salt, and a bit of olive oil, as this helps break down the fibers a bit.

Lemon. This versatile citrus fruit is used for its juice and its zest in both sweet and savory recipes. Lemons are high in the antioxidant vitamin C, which decreases oxidative damage and stress to the body, and is good for overall health and wellness.

Lentils. Lentils come in a variety of colors, each offering its own unique composition of antioxidants and phytochemicals. Lentils are 25 percent protein and an excellent meat alternative. They are a great source of iron, B vitamins, magnesium, zinc, and potassium. They are an excellent choice for optimal brain, cardiovascular, and overall health.

Mint. Mint is a particularly good source of vitamin A. It is also a potent source of antioxidants, especially when compared to other herbs and spices. Antioxidants help protect your body from oxidative stress, a type of damage to cells caused by free radicals. Protecting your body from this damage is one of the best things you can do to stay healthy.

Miso. Miso is fermented soybeans that have been made into a paste. The fermentation process promotes the growth of probiotics, beneficial bacteria that provide a wide array of health benefits, including better digestion, a stronger immune system, and good gut health.

Nutritional yeast. Nutritional yeast is a great source of B12 and other B vitamins, and some trace minerals. It is a complete protein and contains all nine essential amino acids that we need in our diet. Nutritional yeast helps protect against oxidative damage and boost your immunity while adding a delicious umami—a depth of flavor also known as the fifth taste—to your food.

Oats. Oats are among the healthiest grains on earth. They are a great way to boost your brain function and mental energy. Oats are in nature gluten-free and a whole grain, but sometimes processed in plants where cross-contamination can occur, so be sure to check the label if you are severely gluten sensitive. Oats are a great source of important vitamins, minerals, fiber, and antioxidants. Studies have shown that the beta-glucan in oats is effective in reducing cholesterol levels, helps regulate blood sugar, and promotes healthy gut bacteria, all of which contribute to good overall health.

Olive oil. Olive oil is rich in monounsaturated oleic acid, which is considered a good fat linked to better overall brain function. Olive oil stimulates neurogenesis and decreases inflammation with BDNF (brain-derived neurotrophic factor), a type of protein for the brain. Olive oil is loaded with powerful antioxidants, which help reduce your risk of many chronic diseases. It has been part of heart-healthy diets for years, and of course we now know that what's good for the heart is good for the brain. When possible try to buy organic extra-virgin olive oil, which is unrefined and unprocessed.

Onion. Onions are members of the Allium genus of flowering plants that also includes garlic, shallots, leeks, and chives. These vegetables contain many vitamins, minerals, and potent plant compounds that have been shown to promote health and fight disease. Onions are a rich source of fiber and prebiotics, which are necessary for optimal gut health. They are also a wonderful source of powerful antioxidants and thiamine, which helps with mental focus and brain protection.

Oranges. Oranges are a healthy source of fiber, vitamin C, thiamine, folate, and antioxidants and are good for your overall health, memory, and brain health. Although naturally sweet, oranges' low glycemic index is explained by their high polyphenol and fiber content, which moderate the rise in blood sugar when the fruit is eaten whole.

Parsley. Parsley is a versatile herb that can be used fresh or dried. It is nutrient dense, specifically in antioxidants, vitamins A, C, and K, as well as folate. All of these are excellent for good overall brain and heart health, as well as decreasing oxidative stress.

Peaches. Peaches are related to plums, apricots, cherries, and almonds. They are considered a stone fruit, because their flesh surrounds a shell that houses a seed. Peaches are high in fiber, vitamins A, C, and K, as well as potassium, calcium, and magnesium. They are also rich in antioxidants, which help protect your body from disease.

Pomegranate seeds. Often called a "super fruit," pomegranates are among the healthiest foods on the planet, packed with nutrients and powerful plant compounds.

They have a wide range of benefits and may help reduce your risk of various serious illnesses, including heart disease, cancer, arthritis, and other inflammatory conditions. They also can boost your memory and enhance exercise performance. The skin of the pomegranate is thick and inedible, but there are hundreds of edible seeds called arils within. The arils can be eaten whole or pressed into juice.

Pumpkin seeds. Hulled pumpkin seeds, also known as pepitas, are rich in antioxidants, iron, zinc, magnesium, and many other nutrients that help protect against disease and reduce inflammation. Their rich nutrient content provides many health benefits, such as supporting overall brain health and immune function.

Quinoa. Quinoa (KEEN-wah) is another ancient grain. It is gluten-free, high in protein, and one of the few plant foods that contain all nine essential amino acids. It is also high in fiber, magnesium, B vitamins, iron, potassium, calcium, phosphorus, vitamin E, and various beneficial antioxidants. This heart-and brain-healthy tiny seed, rich in fiber, minerals, and antioxidants, is one of the most nutritious foods on the planet.

Sage. Sage belongs to the mint family, alongside other herbs like oregano, rosemary, basil, and thyme. Sage is loaded with antioxidants that are linked to several health benefits, including improved brain function and lower cancer risk. It is also rich in vitamins A and K, as well as thiamine and iron.

Sesame seeds. Sesame seeds are a tiny treasure. A three-tablespoonful serving supplies 12 percent of your required daily fiber, which is vital for good digestive health and therefore overall health. Sesame seeds are a good source of thiamine, niacin, and vitamin B6, which are necessary for proper cellular function and metabolism. Sesame seeds also supply iron and copper, which are needed for blood cell formation and function.

(Tahini, a paste made from grinding toasted sesame seeds, is equally beneficial.)

Shrimp. Shrimp provides selenium, vitamin B12, zinc, and omega-3 fatty acids, all important in proper cell function. In addition, shrimp are rich in the antioxidant astaxanthin, which may be beneficial for brain health. Astaxanthin's anti-inflammatory properties may prevent damage to your brain cells.

Spinach. Spinach is a powerhouse of good nutrition. This leafy green is high in the insoluble fiber needed for good gut health, and therefore good overall health. Spinach is also high in vitamin K and the essential mineral iron. Easy to eat cooked or raw, this is a super green to incorporate into your diet.

Strawberries. These beautiful berries are packed with vitamin C, manganese, and antioxidants that reduce oxidative stress and the risk of many chronic diseases. They contain dietary fibers that feed the good bacteria in your gut and improve digestive health. They are also rich in folate, which is important for proper cell functioning and mood.

Sugar snap peas. Sugar snap peas are a member of the legume family and are actually a cross between snow peas and peas. They are rich in fiber, antioxidants, and vitamins A, C, and K. They are delicious raw or cooked and are a great addition to a healthy diet.

Sunflower seeds. Sunflower seeds are technically the fruits of the sunflower plant. Sunflower seeds have a mild, nutty flavor and a firm but tender texture. They are a wonderful source of healthy fats. They're often roasted to enhance flavor but can be eaten raw. They are high in vitamin E and selenium, which function as antioxidants protecting your body from free radical damage and chronic disease.

Sweet potatoes. Sweet potatoes can be orange, white, or purple, and are high in B vitamins, minerals, antioxidants, and fiber. They are rich in beta-carotene, which decreases inflammation, fights cancer, and boosts the brain's plasticity. They are also usually a major part of the diets of those who live to be over 100 years old.

Thyme. Thyme is an herb from the mint family, but it is much more than an after-thought ingredient to add color to the plate. Thyme is packed with vitamin C and a good source of vitamin A, which are good for neuronal health. This powerful little herb has been used medicinally for centuries.

Tomato. The tomato has been known for years for its benefits to cardiovascular health, and that can be translated to the brain as well. Despite botanically being a fruit, it is generally eaten and prepared like a vegetable. Tomatoes are the major dietary source of the antioxidant lycopene, which has been linked to many health benefits, including reduced risk of heart disease, cancer, and cognitive impairment. They are also a great source of vitamin C, potassium, folate, and vitamin K, all important in overall good health.

Turmeric. Turmeric may be the most effective nutritional supplement in existence. Many studies show that it has major benefits for your body and brain. Turmeric is the ingredient in curry powder responsible for its bright yellow color. Curcumin is the active ingredient in turmeric. It has powerful anti-inflammatory effects and is a strong antioxidant. Unfortunately, curcumin is poorly absorbed into the bloodstream. It helps to consume it with black pepper, which contains piperine, a natural substance that enhances the absorption by 2,000 percent. Turmeric is one of the few foods that we may not be able to eat enough of to reap all its benefits. Taking a daily supplement is a good way to ensure you are getting the proper amounts.

Walnuts. To say that walnuts are nutritious is a bit of an understatement. Walnuts provide healthy fats, fiber, vitamins, and minerals—and that is just the beginning of how they support good health. It may be just a coincidence that the shell of the walnut looks like a tiny brain, but research suggests that this nut may indeed be good for your mind. Studies have found that the nutrients in walnuts, including polyunsaturated fat, polyphenols, and vitamin E, may help reduce oxidative damage and inflammation in your brain. Walnuts also contain ellagic acid, which has been shown to have strong cancer-fighting properties.

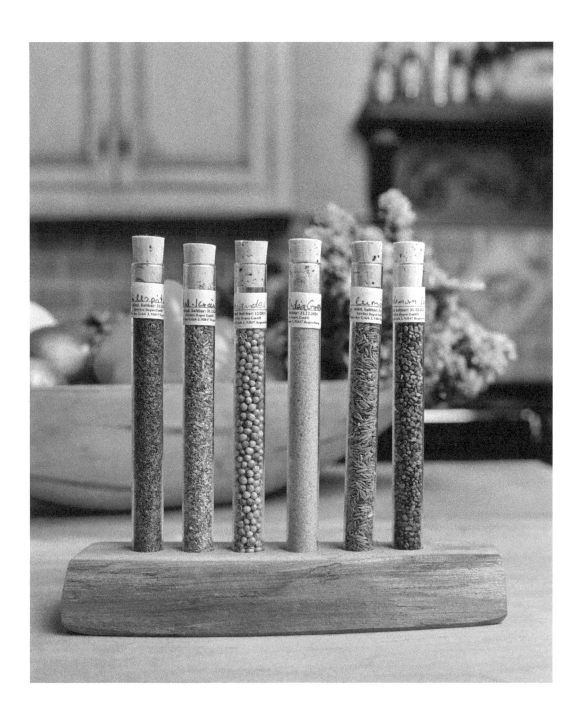

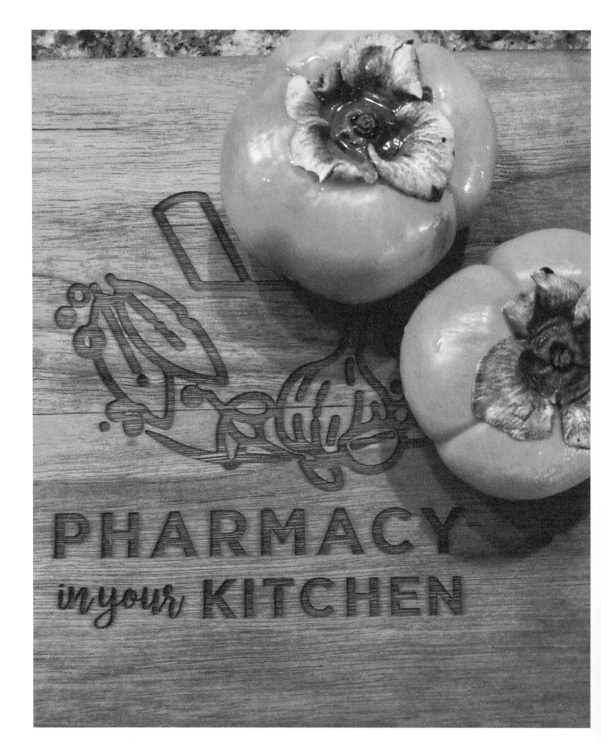

CHAPTER NINETEEN

Recipes

*T*he Pharmacy In Your Kitchen philosophy is really about shifting how you view food and therefore how you choose to eat. There isn't anything magical about any of the recipes that follow. They are merely examples of how to make our dietary recommendations work in your kitchen. Ideally, you will start to look at your own recipes with a new perspective and adapt your favorites to be more in line with what we have suggested below.

BREAKFAST
Baked Blueberry Coconut Oatmeal
Honey Walnut Banana Oat Bread
Tomato, Kale, and Herb Baked Eggs
Overnight Oats with Chia, Carrots, and Raisins
Banana Almond Butter Roll-Ups
Blueberry Walnut Breakfast Cookies
Nutritiously Delicious Granola

SALADS
Healthy Vinaigrette Dressing Seven Ways
Apricot Quinoa Salad
Broccoli Carrot Crunch Salad
Butternut Squash Fall Salad
Triple C Salad
Power Salad with Ancient Grains and Berries
Citrus Salad with Cashews and Pomegranate Seeds
Corn Salad with Black Beans and Farro
Kale and Quinoa Super Salad
Summer Salad with Grilled Peaches and Blueberries

SOUPS
Italian Summer Soup
Lentil Taco Soup
Quick as a Wink Spinach Lentil Soup
Split Pea, Kale, and Carrot Soup
Tuscan White Bean Quinoa Soup

Quinoa Chicken Soup

ADDITIONAL PROTEINS

Rainbow Roasted Eggs

Halibut over Tarragon Lentils and Sweet Potatoes

Maple Glazed Salmon

Shrimp and Grits Reboot with Four Veggies

Shrimp Scampi

EASY MEALS

Rainbow Quinoa "Fried Rice"

Butternut Squash Porter Chili

Sugar Snap Pea and Asparagus Pasta

Pasta Salad with Edamame, Arugula, and Herbs

Salad Pizza

VEGETABLE SIDES

Avocado Strawberry Tomato Salad

Roasted Beets with Citrus and Greens

Kale and Brussels Sprout Caesar Salad

Ginger Miso Slaw

Roasted Butternut Squash with Tahini Dressing and Pomegranate

Roasted Cauliflower and Chickpea Salad

Roasted Root Vegetables with Orange, Ginger, and Turmeric

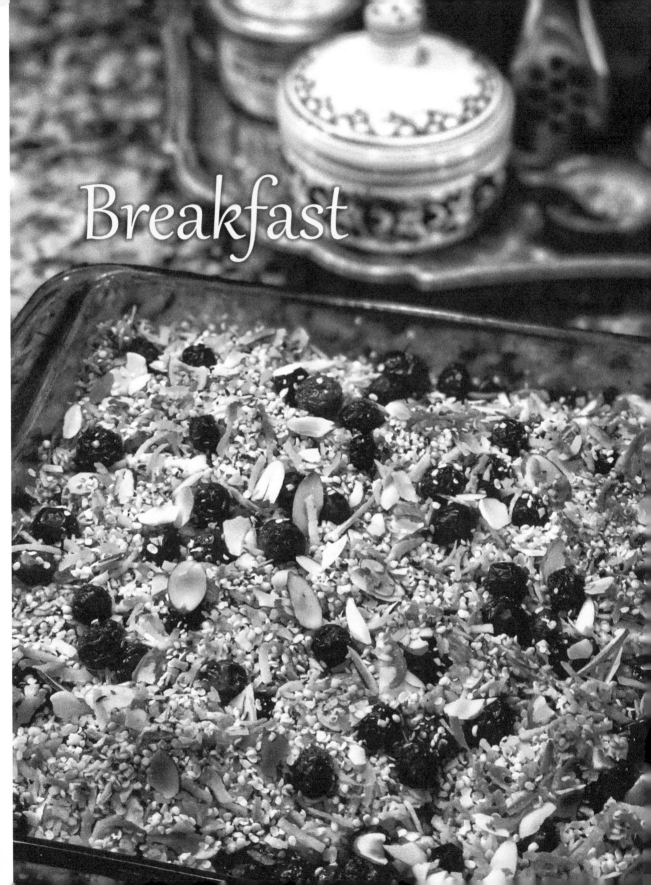

Breakfast

Baked Blueberry Coconut Oatmeal

adapted from *Love and Lemons*

Serves 8

If cobbler and oatmeal had a baby, this nutritious dish is what it would taste like! A delicious way to get the powerful anti-inflammatory benefit of almonds and cinnamon, combined with the antioxidants in the blueberries, all of which improve cognitive function and overall health. The flaxseed is a prebiotic that is good for your gut health, and the hemp seeds are a complete plant-based protein source.

6 Tbsp warm water

2 Tbsp ground flaxseed

½ cup slivered almonds

½ cup hemp seeds (raw and shelled)

⅔ cup unsweetened shredded coconut

2 cups rolled oats

1 tsp baking powder

1 tsp cinnamon

¼ tsp nutmeg

⅛ tsp cardamom

¾ tsp salt

¾ cup unsweetened almond milk

⅓ cup maple syrup

1 tsp vanilla

3 Tbsp melted coconut oil

1 banana, chopped

1½ cups blueberries (divided)

Grease an 8x8-inch baking dish. In a small bowl, combine the flaxseed and water and set aside for at least 5 minutes to thicken. Combine and set aside 2 Tbsp each of the almonds, hemp seeds, and coconut flakes.

continued . . .

163

Baked Blueberry Coconut Oatmeal, continued . . .

In a large bowl, combine the oats, baking powder, spices, salt, and the remaining almonds, hemp seeds, and coconut. In a medium bowl, combine the almond milk, maple syrup, vanilla, coconut oil, and flaxseed/water mixture, and mix well. Pour the wet ingredients into the dry ingredients, and stir to combine.

Layer the banana and 1 cup of the blueberries in the prepared baking dish, and spread the oat mixture on top. Sprinkle with the remaining berries and the reserved almonds, hemp seeds, and coconut.

Bake at 350° for 40–50 minutes, or until a knife inserted in the middle comes out clean. Remove from oven and let cool 15 minutes before serving.

Note: You can halve this recipe and bake for 30 minutes in a 9x5 or similar pan.

Honey Walnut Banana Oat Bread

adapted from *Naturally Nutritious*

Makes 1 loaf

This quick bread has a wonderful texture that resembles that of regular bread. It is slightly sweet, easy to make, and full of brain-boosting nutrition. The oats provide thiamine and magnesium, which improves concentration and mental energy, while the spelt offers magnesium and the added benefit of selenium, which improves memory and cognition. Spelt is a wonderful ancient grain that is much more nutritious than white flour. It is high in fiber and is a delicious way to bump up the nutrition in baking. Spelt provides the excellent texture of this bread; it does, however, contain gluten, which you may react to depending on your gluten sensitivity. And let us not forget to mention the walnuts. Walnuts have strong cancer-fighting properties and are rich in thiamine, vitamin B6, and zinc.

⅓ cup olive oil

½ cup local honey*

2 eggs

¼ cup almond milk

1 tsp vanilla

3 large, very ripe bananas (2 mashed, 1 sliced in half lengthwise)

½ cup rolled oats (plus extra for topping)

1¾ cup spelt flour

2 tsp baking powder

2 tsp cinnamon

pinch of salt

½ cup chopped walnuts

continued . . .

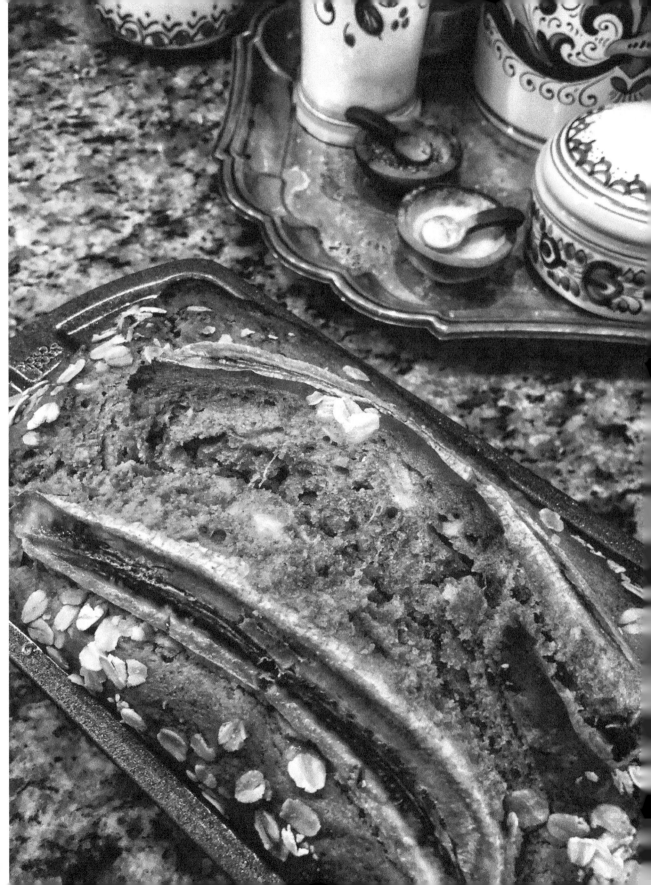

Honey Walnut Banana Oat Bread, continued . . .

In a medium bowl, combine the honey and oil with a whisk. Add the eggs, milk, vanilla, and mashed banana to the bowl and stir to combine. In a larger bowl, combine the oats, flour, baking powder, cinnamon, and salt. Add the wet ingredients to the dry, and gently stir until just combined, being careful not to overmix. Stir in walnuts. Grease a 9x5-inch loaf pan and pour in the prepared batter. Top with banana slices and a few sprinkles of rolled oats.

Bake at 350° for 45–60 minutes or until a wooden skewer inserted in the middle comes out clean. (Be careful not to overbake.) Cool in the pan for 15 minutes, then turn out onto a rack to finish cooling.

*Honey harvested from bees in your area may help build an immunity to some seasonal allergies.

Tomato, Kale, and Herb Baked Eggs

adapted from *The Roasted Root*

Serves 2

This easy and versatile dish can be served for brunch or dinner, and reheats well if there are any leftovers. It offers a rainbow of nutrient-rich colors, and the thyme, parsley and tomatoes provide vitamin A, which helps maintain brain health and cognitive function. The addition of kale, a super green rich in nutrients and fiber, makes this a delicious way to nourish your body any time of day.

3 Tbsp olive oil
4 cups chopped kale
½ tsp red pepper flakes
1 cup cherry or grape tomatoes, halved
4 eggs at room temperature
¼ cup grated Parmesan cheese
2 tsp fresh minced parsley
½ tsp fresh minced thyme
salt and pepper

In a large ovenproof skillet, heat the olive oil over medium heat. Add the kale and red pepper flakes, and sauté until the kale is wilted but not thoroughly cooked. Add the tomatoes and stir to combine. Make 4 wells in the mixture and crack a whole egg in each. In a small bowl, combine the cheese, parsley, and thyme, and then sprinkle on top of the egg and kale mixture. Season with salt and pepper.

Bake at 350° for 6–8 minutes, or until the eggs are done as you prefer.

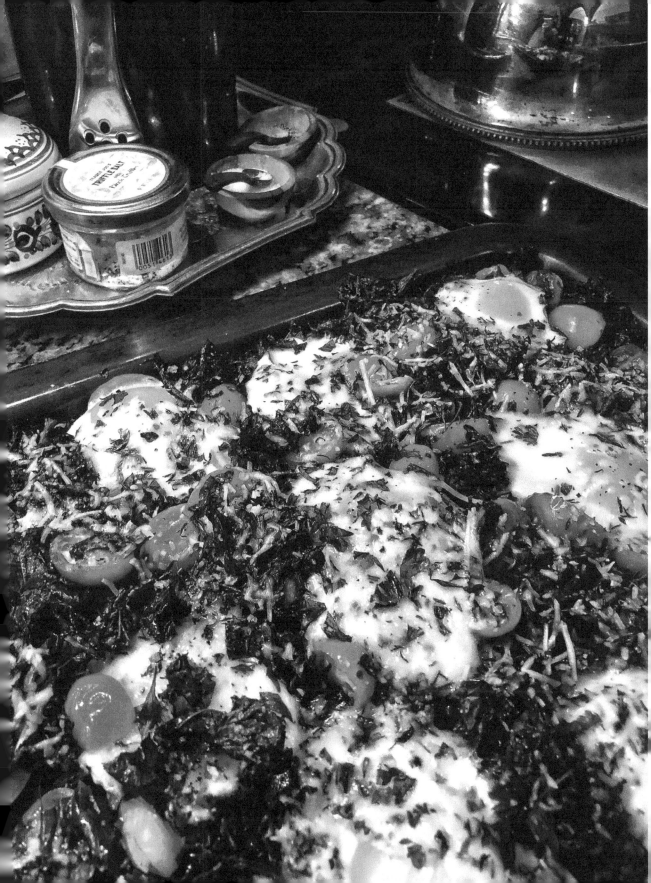

Overnight Oats with Chia, Carrots, and Raisins

adapted from *The Roasted Root*

Serves 6

This is an easy make-ahead breakfast packed with nutrition. The chia seeds are full of antioxidants and omega-3 ALA, used to make fatty acids, that are necessary for good brain function. The carrots provide both memory-enhancing vitamin K and vitamin A, which helps the aging brain. Finally, the walnuts bring plant protein and cancer-fighting nutrients to start your day off right.

> 4 cups unsweetened almond milk
>
> 2 cups rolled oats
>
> 1 cup grated carrot
>
> ⅔ cup raisins
>
> ⅓ cup chopped walnuts
>
> ½ cup unsweetened shredded coconut
>
> 3 Tbsp maple syrup
>
> 2 Tbsp chia seeds
>
> 1 tsp cinnamon
>
> ½ tsp nutmeg
>
> ⅛ tsp cardamom

In a large mixing bowl, stir all ingredients until well combined.

Cover and refrigerate overnight.

Before serving, stir and top with some almond butter if desired.

Store covered and sealed in the refrigerator for up to 5 days.

Banana Almond Butter Roll-Ups

by Pharmacy In Your Kitchen

Serves 1

This is my husband's favorite quick and nutritious breakfast. So easy to make, but such a great way to start the day. The almond butter is anti-inflammatory (unlike peanut butter, which actually causes inflammation), and the banana provides vitamin B6, a memory enhancer; magnesium, which facilitates electrical activity in your brain's nerve cells; and tryptophan and tyrosine, needed to make serotonin and dopamine, which keep you calm and focused and stabilize your mood.

> 1 flour tortilla (ancient grain is best)
> 1–2 Tbsp almond butter
> 1 banana

Warm the tortilla in an ungreased large skillet over medium heat until it just starts to brown. Flip and repeat on the other side. Remove from pan and spread with almond butter. Place the banana at one edge of the tortilla and roll up. Slice into bite-sized rolls.

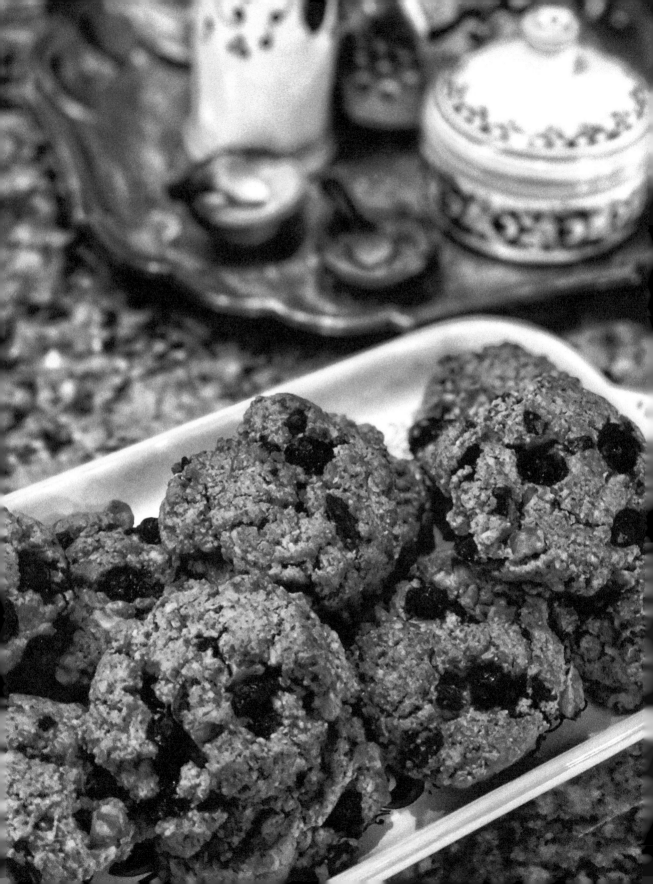

Blueberry Walnut Breakfast Cookies

adapted from *Love and Lemons*

Makes 12

I almost didn't call these cookies, but I thought it would show that you can have fun and eat well at the same time. Instead of bleached and processed white flour, it uses the nutritional powerhouses of oats (as flour and rolled) and almonds (as flour and almond butter). The almonds and oats are also good examples of "heart healthy" foods that are also good for your brain. So while you are improving your cognitive function, you are actually taking good care of your heart and whole body. Additionally, the blueberry and goji berries provide many health benefits, including cancer protection and antioxidants. Well done for a cookie!

- 5 Tbsp warm water
- 2 Tbsp ground flaxseed
- 1 cup oat flour
- 1 cup rolled oats
- ½ cup almond flour
- 1 tsp cinnamon
- ½ tsp baking powder
- ½ tsp baking soda
- ½ tsp nutmeg
- ¼ tsp cardamom
- ½ tsp salt
- zest of a large lemon
- ½ cup almond butter
- ½ cup maple syrup
- ¼ cup coconut oil melted
- ½ cup walnuts, chopped
- 3 Tbsp dried goji berries (optional)
- ¾ cup blueberries

continued . . .

Blueberry Walnut Breakfast Cookies, continued . . .

In a small bowl, combine the flaxseed and water and set aside.

In a large bowl, combine the dry ingredients and the lemon zest.

In a separate bowl, combine the almond butter, maple syrup, and coconut oil, and stir until smooth. Stir the flaxseed mixture into the liquids. Add the wet ingredients to the dry and mix until just combined. Add the walnuts and goji berries and stir again, being careful not to overmix. Add the blueberries and fold in gently to prevent crushing the blueberries. Place ¼ cup of the mixture onto a parchment-lined cookie sheet and repeat for 12 cookies.

Bake at 350° for 20 minutes until browned on the edges. Remove from the oven, let sit on cookie sheet for 5 minutes to set, then transfer to a cooling rack.

Nutritiously Delicious Granola

adapted from Heidi Schulz

Makes 6 cups

This is an easy and delicious breakfast or snack that will make your kitchen smell amazing! The oats give you more mental energy, while the cinnamon provides anti-inflammatory benefits for the brain and your whole body. Walnuts are memory boosters, cancer fighters, and an overall incredible nut to add to your diet. Although you could use any dried fruit you like, I use organic cherries because they provide powerful antioxidants, they are cancer fighting, and they're full of melatonin, which helps you get a good night's sleep.

4 cups rolled oats
1 cup chopped walnuts
1 cup dried cherries (unsweetened if possible)
¼ cup unsweetened shredded coconut
1 tsp cinnamon
¼ tsp nutmeg
1/8 tsp cardamom
½ tsp salt
5 Tbsp melted coconut oil
2 egg whites, lightly beaten
⅓ cup maple syrup
1 tsp vanilla

In a large bowl, mix together oats, walnuts, cherries, coconut, spices, and salt. In a smaller bowl, whisk together the remaining ingredients. Pour wet ingredients into dry and stir well. Spread evenly onto a very large rimmed baking sheet lined with parchment paper, and make a donut sized hole in the middle to allow everything to cook evenly.

Bake for 25–35 minutes in a 300° oven. DO NOT STIR while baking, and cool for 15 minutes before breaking into clumps.

If there are any leftovers, transfer to an airtight jar to store.

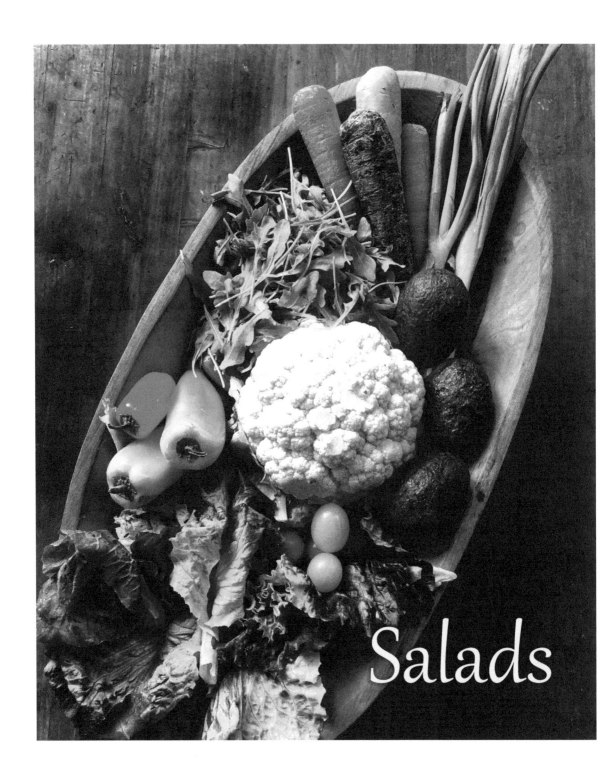

Salads

Healthy Vinaigrette Dressing Seven Ways

by Pharmacy In Your Kitchen

Store-bought salad dressings can be packed with unhealthy ingredients like added sugar and saturated fats. Making your own vinaigrette is quick and easy and so much better for you. This basic recipe—with the cancer-fighting, cardiovascular, brain-health benefits of garlic—can be used as is, or you can add a few things for some variety of flavor and other health benefits.

Basic Vinaigrette

3 Tbsp red wine vinegar

1 garlic clove, minced

1 tsp Dijon mustard

¾ tsp salt

pepper to taste

¾ cup extra virgin olive oil

Combine all ingredients in a small mason jar or other covered glass jar. Shake to blend.

Greek Vinaigrette

Basic Vinaigrette PLUS:

1 tsp dried oregano (enhances memory, mood, and motivation)

½ tsp lemon zest

Miso Vinaigrette

Basic Vinaigrette PLUS:

1 Tbsp white miso paste (naturally fermented soybeans, great for gut health)

continued . . .

French Vinaigrette

Basic Vinaigrette PLUS:

1 tsp dried tarragon (has manganese, good for brain health)

Spicy Sesame Vinaigrette

Basic Vinaigrette PLUS:

1 Tbsp toasted sesame seeds (improves memory)

1 Tbsp toasted sesame oil

1 tsp crushed red pepper

Kimchi Vinaigrette

Basic Vinaigrette PLUS:

2 Tbsp finely chopped Kimchi cabbage (naturally fermented spicy cabbage, great for gut health)

Ginger Vinaigrette

Basic Vinaigrette PLUS:

2 Tbsp peeled and grated fresh ginger (increases ability to focus)

Apricot Quinoa Salad

adapted from *Love and Lemons*

Serves 4

I love fresh apricots, but you don't usually see a salad recipe using them. When in season, I love adding them to this salad, as they are rich in vitamins A and C and full of antioxidants. The memory-boosting quinoa mixed with cumin and the healthy fats of the avocado make for a wonderful and seasonal salad that will not disappoint. 3 cups mixed greens

1 cup cooked quinoa

1 cup canned chickpeas, drained and rinsed

3 cups mixed greens

1 avocado, cubed

½ cup fresh apricots, diced

¼ cup almonds, toasted and chopped

¼ cup chopped chives

Dressing:

¼ cup olive oil

2 cloves garlic, minced

juice of 1 lemon

2 tsp honey

2 tsp cumin

salt and pepper

In a large bowl, toss together the greens, quinoa, chickpeas, avocado, and apricots. In a small bowl, whisk together dressing ingredients. Drizzle the salad mixture with dressing to your taste (save remainder for other salads). Top with toasted almonds and chives. Season with salt and pepper.

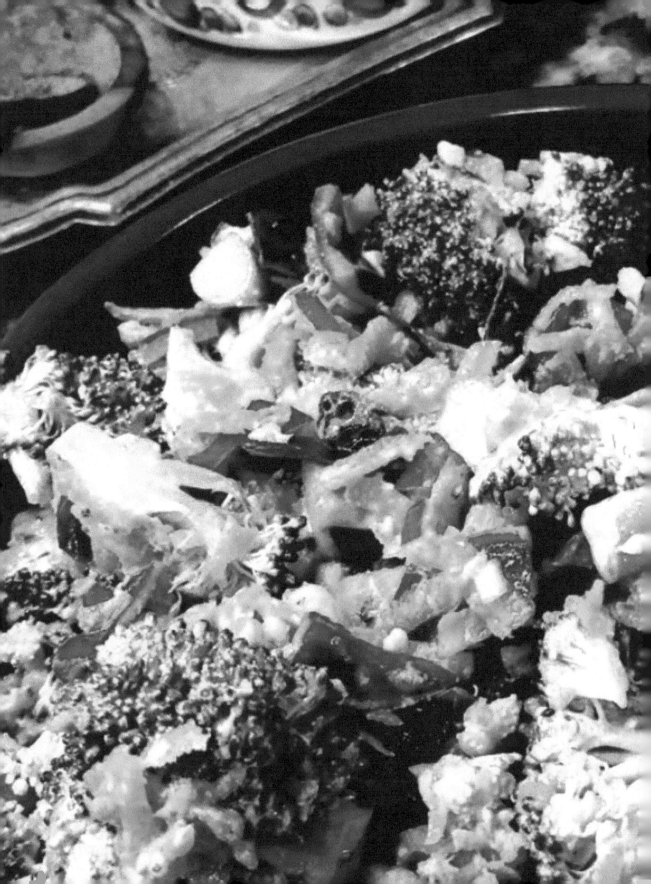

Broccoli Carrot Crunch Salad

adapted from *Functional Foods*

Serves 4

This salad is loaded with vitamins A, K, and C, calcium, and fiber. It uses the cruciferous powerhouse foods—broccoli and cabbage—which are known cancer-fighting vegetables. While it is delicious the day you make it, it tastes even better the next day, making it ideal for meal prepping. This salad promotes healthy brain function and overall good health.

1 large head of broccoli florets, chopped

1½ cups grated carrots (use as many different colors as you can find)

1 cup chopped red cabbage

¼ cup diced red onions

¼ cup chopped roasted cashews

¼ cup raisins

Dressing:

6 Tbsp Dijon mustard

½ cup unsweetened almond milk

2½ Tbsp apple cider vinegar

2 Tbsp olive oil

1 clove garlic minced

salt and pepper

In a large bowl, combine the broccoli, carrots, cabbage, onion, cashews, and raisins. In a smaller bowl, whisk together the dressing ingredients. Toss the salad with some of the dressing (save remainder for later use). Season with salt and pepper to taste.

Butternut Squash Fall Salad

adapted from *Love and Lemons*

Serves 4

There are so many wonderful fruits and vegetables in the fall, and this salad showcases some of my favorites. The butternut squash is rich in color, fiber, and phytonutrients, and I love using it in a salad. The dressing uses the natural sweetness of dates, and a small amount of goat cheese adds a wonderful flavor; since it has a different protein than cow's milk, it is easier to digest. Top it off with pistachios and pomegranate seeds, and this salad will keep you focused all day!

1 butternut squash, peeled, seeded, and cubed

1 Tbsp olive oil

¼ tsp ground cumin

¼ tsp ground coriander

¼ tsp cinnamon

¼ tsp cayenne pepper

4 cups salad greens of choice

2 cups sliced cabbage

2 Medjool dates, pitted and diced

¼ cup pomegranate seeds

¼ cup pistachios, chopped

salt and pepper

2 oz goat cheese, crumbled

continued . . .

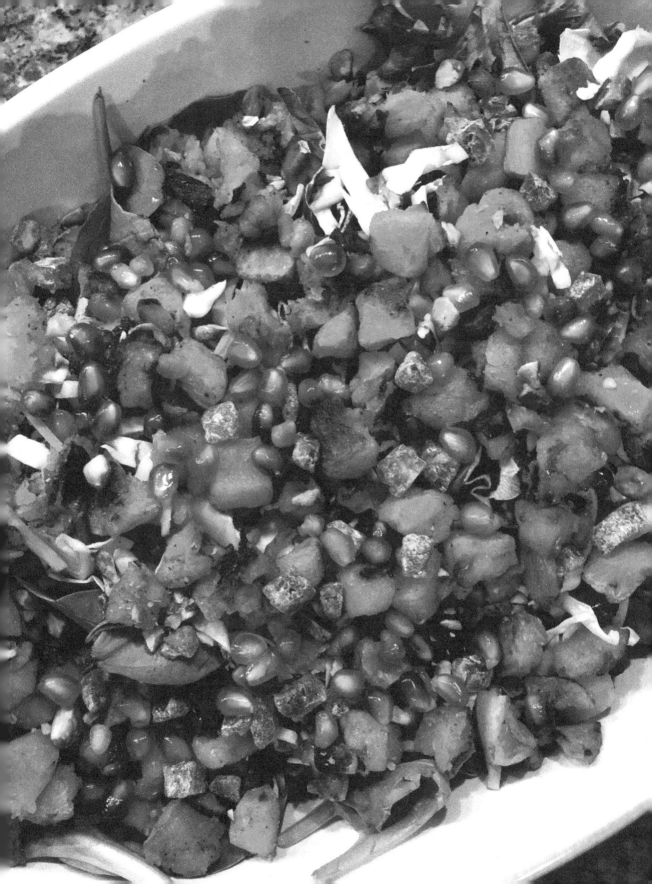

Dressing:
5 Tbsp olive oil
4 Tbsp water
3 Tbsp apple cider vinegar
1 Medjool date, pitted
1 small clove of garlic, minced
⅛ tsp ground cumin
¼ tsp salt

Place the butternut squash on a large baking sheet lined with parchment paper. Drizzle 1 Tbsp olive oil over the squash, toss, and season with salt and pepper. Bake at 450° for 25–30 minutes or until tender and browned around the edges. Set aside to cool slightly.

In a small bowl, mix the cumin, coriander, cinnamon, and cayenne, and set aside. Once the squash is cooled, toss it with the spice mixture.

Combine greens, cabbage, and squash in a large bowl.

In a blender, mix the dressing ingredients. Toss salad with about half the dressing, or to taste. Then add the remaining dates, pomegranates, and pistachios, and lightly toss. Drizzle with more dressing if desired. Add crumbled goat cheese, if desired, and serve immediately.

Triple C Salad with Couscous, Cherries, and Chickpeas

adapted from *Pinch of Yum*

Serves 4

This salad uses couscous as a base because it is high in selenium and B6, both of which support good brain health. The chickpeas are high in folate and magnesium, the cherries are full of antioxidants, and the addition of all the wonderful spices make this dish an easy winner.

1¼ cups chicken stock
1 tsp ground cumin
1 tsp ground coriander
1 cup uncooked couscous
½ cup dried cherries (preferably unsweetened)
¼ cup diced red onion
salt and pepper
8 oz canned chickpeas, drained
2 cups baby spinach, roughly chopped
1 avocado, cubed
½ cup roasted salted sunflower seeds

Dressing:
½ cup olive oil
¼ cup fresh-squeezed lemon juice
1 Tbsp honey
¼ cup chopped parsley
¼ cup chopped mint
salt and pepper

In a saucepan, bring stock, cumin, and coriander to a boil. Add the couscous, cover, and remove from heat. After 5 minutes, fluff with a fork, and transfer to a serving bowl. Add the cherries and red onion, fluff again, and let cool. Whisk together dressing ingredients. When the couscous is cool, add the dressing a little at a time until it is nicely flavored, but not too wet. Save remainder to use as a marinade or dressing for another salad). When ready to serve, gently toss in the chickpeas, spinach, avocado, and seeds.

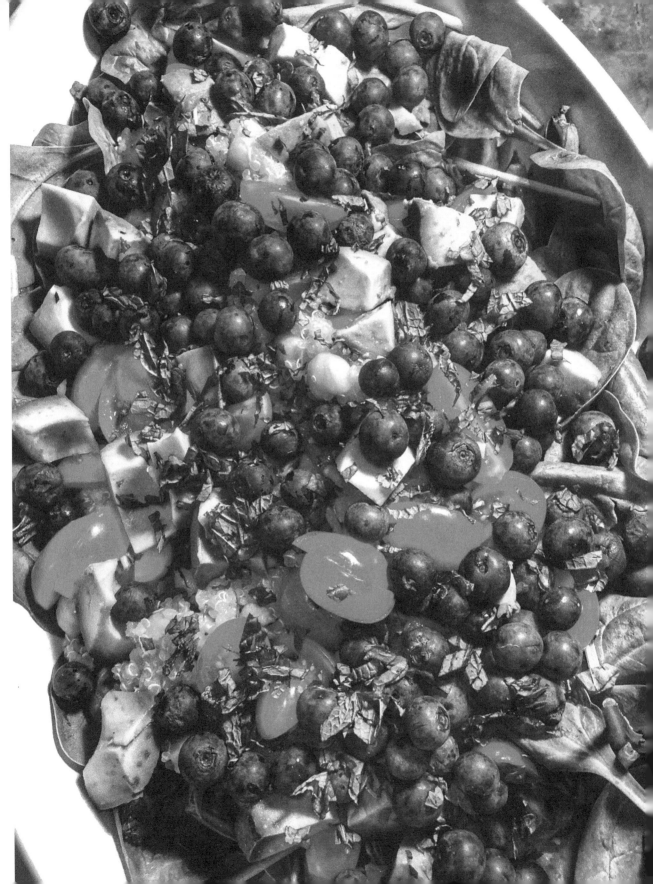

Power Salad with Ancient Grains and Berries

adapted from *Cooking Light*

Serves 4

This is my favorite salad to stay alert and avoid the post-lunch slump. The ancient grain of quinoa is not only high in protein, but also zinc and folate, which keep our memories strong and brains healthy. The tomatoes are rich in vitamins A and B, and antioxidants that improve cognitive function and reduce the risk for heart disease and cancer. The sunflower seeds are not only a tasty addition of protein, but also decrease inflammation and cognitive decline. Finally, the lemon is rich in folate, which has memory-boosting flavonoids and makes the salad taste fresh and light.

Dressing:
¼ cup olive oil
¼ cup apple cider vinegar
2 Tbsp fresh lemon juice
1 Tbsp local honey
1½ tsp poppy seeds
1 tsp minced shallot
½ tsp salt
black pepper to taste

1 cup canned chickpeas, rinsed and drained
1 cup cooked quinoa (or other ancient grain, like farro)
4 cups packed fresh baby spinach (or other dark salad green)
1 cup organic blueberries (or other berry or seasonal stone fruit)
1 cup halved grape tomatoes
2 Tbsp roasted salted sunflower seeds
1 avocado, cubed
2 oz crumbled sheep's milk feta or goat cheese (optional)
2 Tbsp chopped mint leaves

Whisk together dressing ingredients. Combine chickpeas and ancient grain in a large bowl. Add 3 Tbsp dressing and toss to combine. Add remaining ingredients and toss with remaining dressing

Citrus Salad with Cashews and Pomegranate Seeds

adapted from *Martha Stewart*

Serves 4

This winter salad is bursting with color and wonderful nutrition. When citrus is in season, take advantage of all this beautiful dish has to offer. The grapefruit and oranges provide vitamins A and C, which are good for cardiovascular and brain health. The cashews provide protein and zinc, thiamine, and vitamin E. Finally, topping it all off are the beautiful and delicious pomegranate seeds, which have been called a super fruit for their many health benefits, including reducing the risk for heart disease, cancer, and inflammatory diseases.

    2 grapefruits, peeled and sliced, slices halved
    2 oranges, peeled and sliced
    2 kiwifruit, peeled and sliced
    ¼ cup toasted cashews, chopped
    ¼ cup chopped mint leaves
    ½ cup pomegranate seeds

Arrange sliced fruit on a serving platter. Pour any extra juices that you may have leftover on top of the fruit. Top with cashews, mint, and pomegranate seeds. Lightly sprinkle with salt if desired.

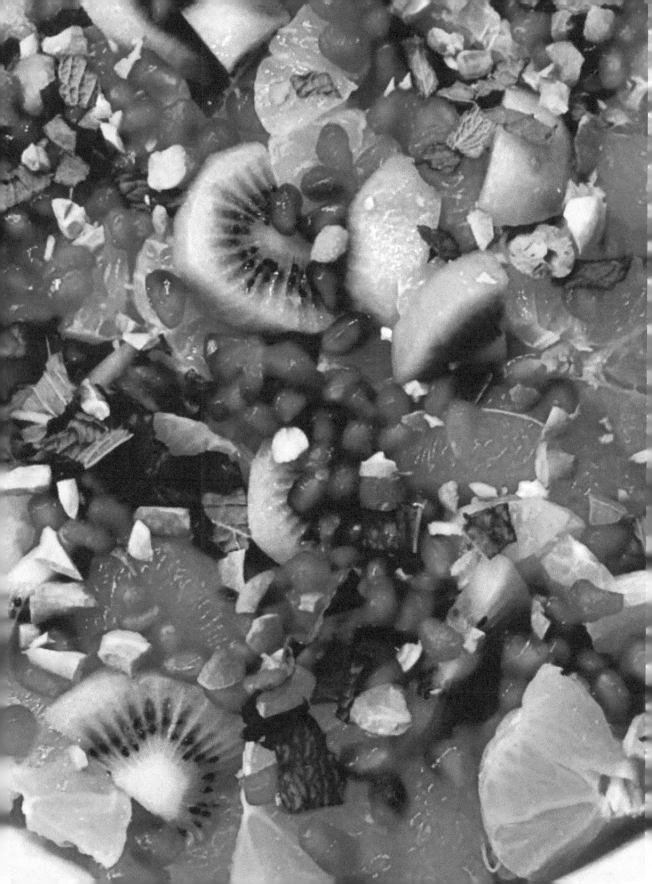

Corn Salad with Black Beans and Farro

adapted from *Eating Well*

Serves 4

This wonderful salad comes together easily with the help of the canned beans and prepared salsa. It uses the ancient grain farro, which is high in fiber and protein and full of B vitamins that are good for overall brain health (though if you have gluten sensitivity, you can replace the cooked farro with cooked quinoa). The beans and the healthy fat in the avocado add the benefit of decreasing inflammation, which is good for your entire body, including your brain. Finally, the cumin improves cognitive function and adds a wonderful flavor to the dish.

2 cups water
1 tsp salt
1 cup farro, rinsed and drained
15-oz can black beans, drained and rinsed
1 Tbsp olive oil
3 ears of corn, kernels cut off cobs
½ red onion, chopped
salt and pepper
1 avocado, peeled and diced

Dressing:
½ cup salsa (plus extra for topping)
½ cup fresh-squeezed orange juice
⅓ cup fresh-squeezed lime juice
3 Tbsp chopped cilantro
1 Tbsp olive oil
¾ tsp ground cumin
salt and pepper

In a large saucepan, bring water and salt to a boil. Add the rinsed farro, reduce heat, and simmer for 20 minutes, or until all the water is absorbed. Transfer to a large bowl.

In a large skillet, sauté the corn and onions in 1 Tbsp olive oil. Season with salt and pepper to taste, and cook until tender and browned. Add this mixture and the rinsed beans to the farro.

In a small bowl, combine salsa, orange juice, lime juice, cilantro, oil, cumin, salt, and pepper. Toss with the farro mixture. Top with avocado and a few spoonfuls of salsa.

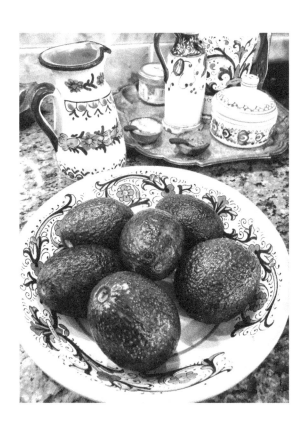

Kale and Quinoa Super Salad

adapted from The Roasted Root

I call this a super salad because it has three ingredients that get a lot of attention for their nutritional value. First, kale is called a super green because it is loaded with powerful nutrition that your body and brain need to stay healthy and strong. Quinoa is an ancient grain high in protein and also great for overall health. Finally, hemp seeds offer more plant-based protein, and are rich in antioxidants as well. Combine them with the anti-inflammatory benefits of the apples and walnuts, and the magnesium in the pumpkin seeds, then toss them in a healthy oil and fresh lemon juice, and you have a salad loaded with optimal nutrition. Serves 2

> 2 bunches lacinato kale (Tuscan or dinosaur kale), chopped
> fresh lemon juice
> ⅔ cup cooked quinoa
> ½ apple, thinly sliced
> ¼ cup walnuts, toasted
> ¼ cup pumpkin seeds, toasted
> 3 Tbsp dried cranberries
> 1 Tbsp hemp seeds
> avocado oil (may substitute olive oil)
> salt and pepper

In a large bowl, drizzle 2 Tbsp of lemon juice over the chopped kale. Use your hands to massage the kale until it starts to soften. (This usually takes several minutes; the kale becomes more pliable and takes up less room in the bowl.) Let stand for 10 minutes. Add remaining ingredients to the kale with more oil, lemon juice, and salt and pepper to taste. Toss well to combine.

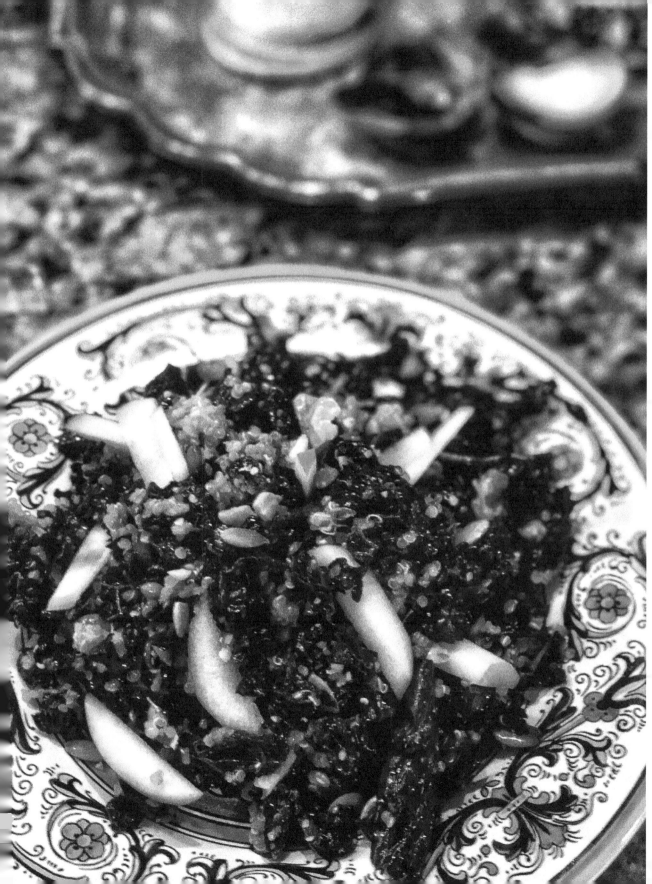

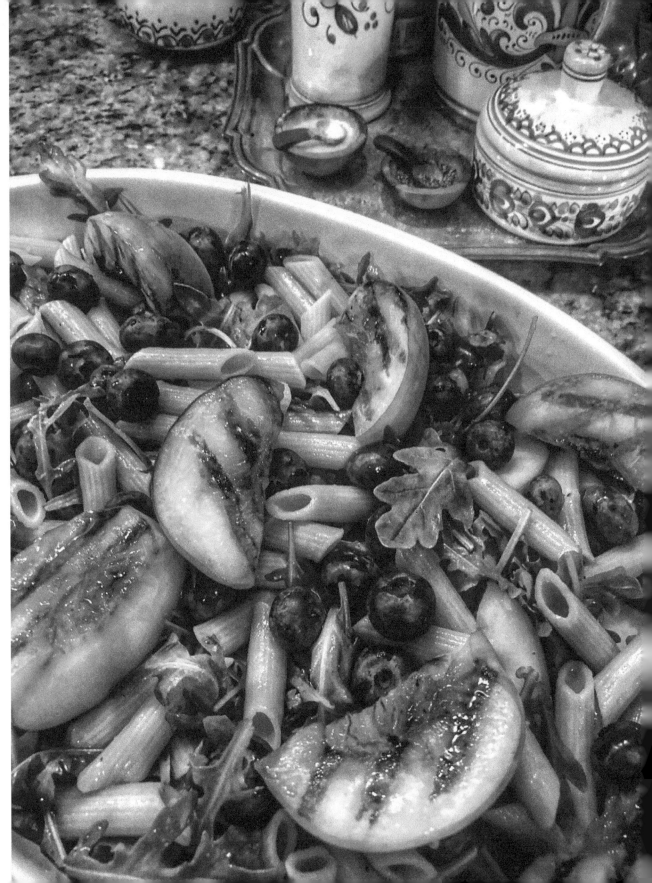

Summer Salad with Grilled Peaches and Blueberries

adapted from *Forks Over Knives*

Serves 6

This summer salad is gorgeous and nutritious. It takes advantage of seasonal peaches and blueberries and combines them with a healthy ancient-grain pasta*, spicy arugula, and a simple dressing. Grilling the peaches gives a wonderful sweetness to this dish; this can be done on a traditional grill or with a grill pan on the stove.

4 cups dry ancient-grain penne pasta

4 firm, ripe peaches, halved and pitted

5 oz fresh arugula

2 cups fresh blueberries

Dressing:

¾ cup olive oil

½ cup fresh-squeezed lemon juice

4 tsp Dijon mustard

4 cloves garlic, minced

1 Tbsp maple syrup

1 tsp lemon zest

salt and pepper

Cook pasta according to package directions. Drain and set aside to cool.

Place the peach halves cut side down on a hot traditional grill or on a stove using a greased grill pan that is very hot. Cook about 8 minutes, or until desired grill marks appear. Remove from heat and allow to cool. Cut peach halves into quarters and set aside.

In a small bowl, make the dressing by whisking together the olive oil, lemon juice, mustard, garlic, maple syrup, and lemon zest. Season with salt and pepper to taste.

continued . . .

In a large bowl or salad platter, combine the pasta, arugula, blueberries, and peaches, and toss with some of the dressing as desired. Save the remaining dressing for other salads and marinades.

Note: This salad holds up well for at least an hour after it is dressed, so it can be made ahead if desired.

*In this recipe, I used ancient grain pasta, but you could use a bean or lentil pasta or your personal favorite. Typically, I don't use a wheat pasta because ancient grains have a higher nutritional value and are non-GMO and unbleached.

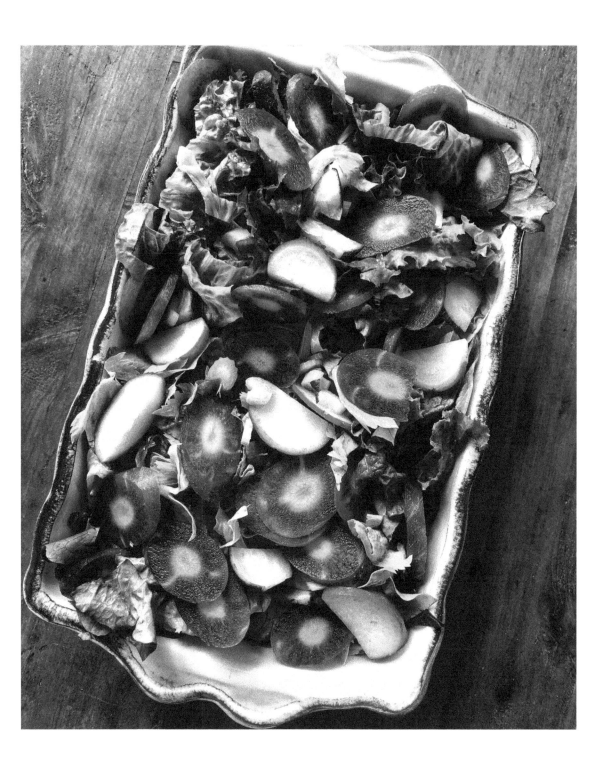

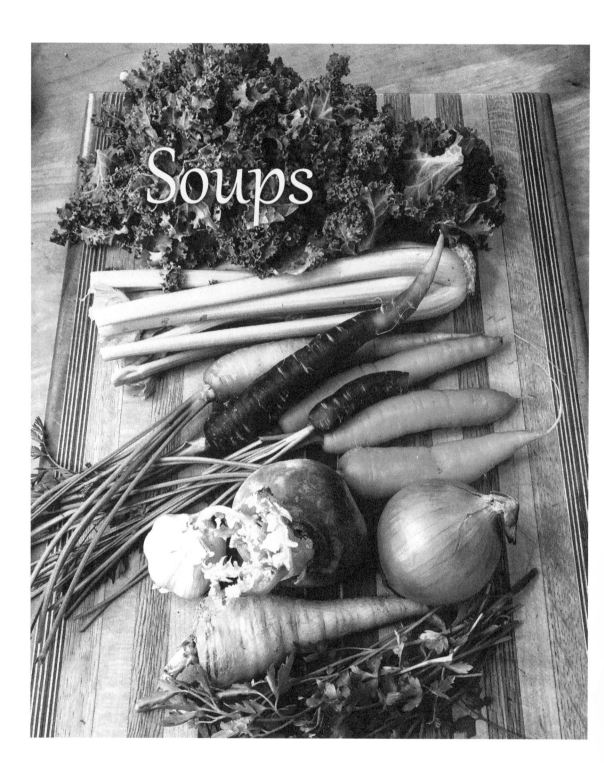

Soups

Italian Summer Soup

adapted from Pinch of Yum

Serves 8

This delicious soup is full of the beautiful colors of summer and comes together very quickly for those busy summer days. As with most soups, it is wonderful the day it is made but gets even better the next day as a lunch or leftover supper. The beans are a great way to get protein while avoiding or decreasing the meat in your diet, and they add a very satisfying creaminess to the soup. This soup calls for both fresh and dried onions and garlic. The addition of the dried varieties boosts the flavor and nutritional value of two of my favorite healthful ingredients.

2 Tbsp olive oil

½ cup diced yellow onion

4 carrots, chopped

2 stalks of celery, chopped

3 cloves of garlic, minced

6 cups chicken or vegetable broth

1 28-oz can crushed tomatoes

1 16-oz can cannellini beans, drained

¾ cup uncooked farro

1 tsp dried basil

1 tsp dried oregano

½ tsp garlic powder

½ tsp onion powder

2 tsp salt

2 medium zucchini, diced

3 cups fresh corn kernels, cut off the cob

fresh chopped parsley to garnish

In a soup pot over medium heat, warm the olive oil and sauté the onions, carrots, celery, and garlic until tender. Add the broth, tomatoes, beans, farro, basil, oregano, garlic and onion powders, and salt, and bring to a boil. Cover and simmer 20 minutes. Add zucchini and corn and simmer an additional 5 minutes or until tender. Garnish with fresh parsley if desired.

Lentil Taco Soup

adapted from *The Garden Grazer*

Serves 4

This soup originally didn't have kale or any grains in it, and you can certainly make it without them if you prefer. But I thought it needed a bit more color and heartiness, so I added both. Adding kale to just about anything is one of the healthiest things you can do in your diet, so I sneak it in whenever I can. Soup is an easy way to add beans and lentils into your meals, and the combination in this recipe offers a double hit of B vitamins and minerals your body needs. As for adding the grains, I typically just add whatever rice or pasta I have left over from the night before to bulk it up a bit. I prefer the ancient grains and darker rices, as they are higher in fiber and nutrients than white grains.

    2 Tbsp olive oil
    1 yellow onion, diced
    3 cloves garlic, minced
    3 Tbsp taco seasoning*
    4 cups chicken or vegetable broth
    1 cup dry brown lentils, rinsed and drained
    1 15-oz can diced tomatoes
    3 cups shredded kale
    1 15-oz can black beans, rinsed and drained
    1 cup corn (fresh or frozen)
    1 cup cooked ancient grain pasta (or rice)

    Optional garnishes:
    avocado, diced
    green onions, sliced
    fresh cilantro or Italian parsley, chopped
    shredded cheese of choice
    hot sauce

continued . . .

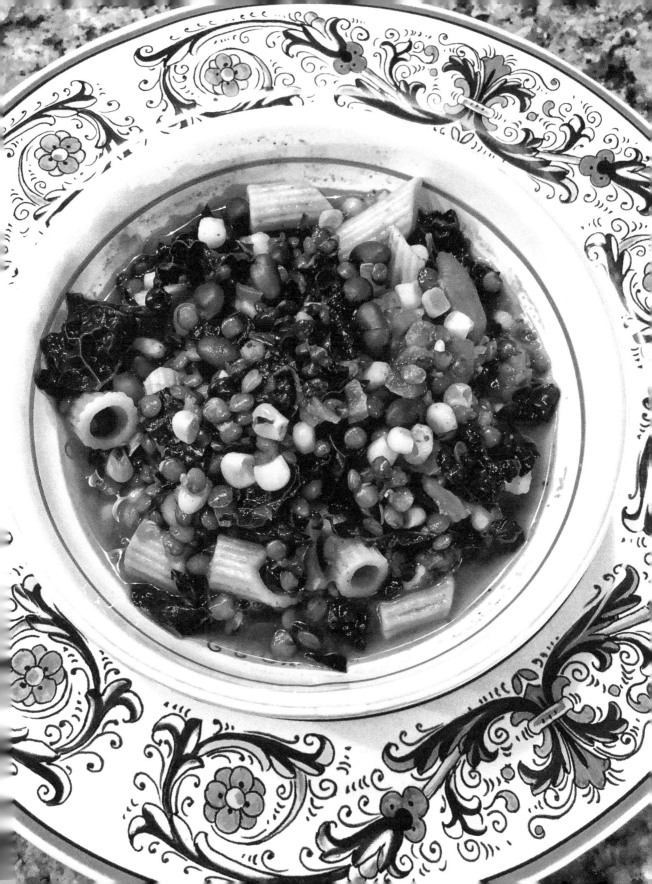

Lentil Taco Soup, continued . . .

In a soup pot, warm the olive oil over medium heat. Add the onion and sauté until tender, then add in the garlic and taco seasoning and cook a minute longer. Add the broth, lentils, tomatoes, and kale, and bring to a boil. Reduce heat, cover, and simmer for 30 minutes. Stir in the beans, corn, and grains, and cook for additional 5–10 minutes or until desired tenderness. To serve, ladle into bowls and garnish as desired.

Homemade Taco Seasoning:
1 Tbsp chili powder
1½ tsp cumin
1 tsp oregano
1 tsp onion powder
1 tsp garlic powder
1 tsp paprika
½ tsp salt
Combine all ingredients. Store in an airtight container.

Quick as a Wink Spinach Lentil Soup

by Pharmacy In Your Kitchen

Serves 6

This is one of those recipes that comes together quickly, yet tastes like it took hours to make! We need options like this so that we can eat well and nourish our bodies simply. Pull this one out when you need to do just that! It combines the powerful team of garlic and onions with Asian mushrooms, spinach, thyme, and sage to make a delicious and very nutritious immune-boosting soup rich in vitamins A, C, and K for optimal health and brain function.

2 Tbsp olive oil

½ yellow onion, diced

3 cloves garlic, minced

1 carrot, peeled and chopped

1 stalk of celery, chopped

4 oz mushrooms, chopped (I like shiitake and other Asian varieties)

1 tsp dried thyme

½ tsp dried sage

½ tsp salt

½ tsp pepper

2 cups stock or broth of choice

1 15-oz can green lentils, drained and rinsed (or 2 cups cooked lentils)

1 15-oz can black-eyed peas, drained and rinsed (or 2 cups cooked black-eyed peas)

1 14-oz can coconut milk

1 Tbsp apple cider vinegar

1 Tbsp soy sauce

5 oz fresh spinach, chopped

continued . . .

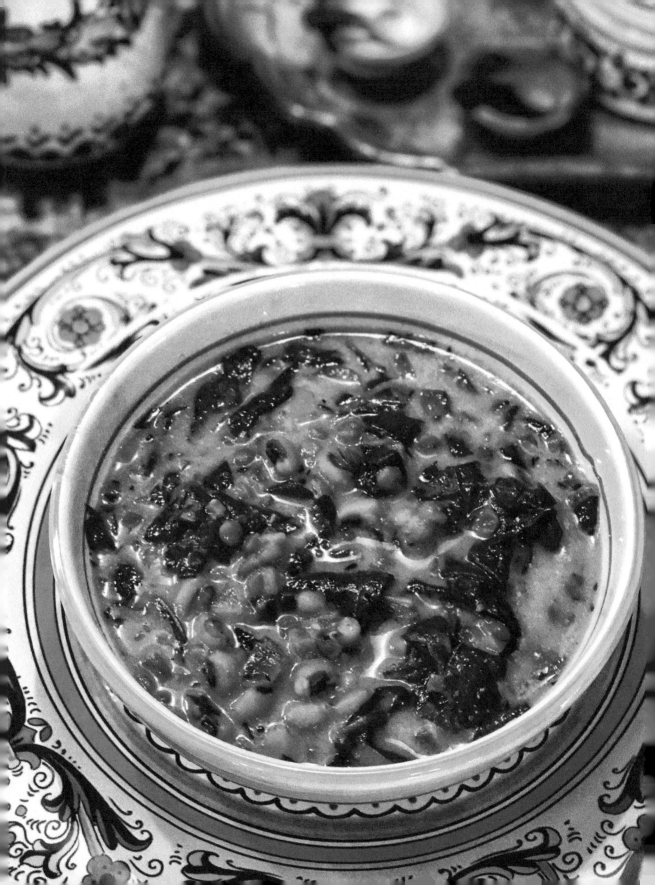

In a stockpot, heat the oil over medium heat. Add the onion and cook until soft and translucent. Next, add the garlic, carrot, and celery, and sauté a few minutes more, being careful not to burn. Add the mushrooms, thyme, sage, salt, and pepper. Cook for 5 more minutes then add the broth or stock, lentils, black-eyed peas, coconut milk, vinegar, and soy sauce. Simmer 10 minutes, and then add the spinach to wilt. Season with salt and pepper to taste. Serve immediately, or remove from heat so as to not overcook the spinach.

Split Pea, Kale, and Carrot Soup

adapted from *Feed Me Phoebe*

Serves 4–6

This soup is so delicious that I recommend you try it even if you don't particularly like peas or kale! I make it a little less pureed than typical pea soup so I can recognize the vegetables, but that is a personal preference. Not only does this recipe contain some of my favorite veggies, but it also uses curry, which is a nutritional powerhouse. Curry is a mixture of turmeric, cumin, coriander, ginger, chilies, and several other wonderful spices that offer cancer-fighting, anti-inflammatory, and brain-boosting nutrition.

> 3 Tbsp olive oil
> 2 carrots, diced
> 1 onion, diced
> 2 cups very finely chopped kale
> 2 cloves garlic, minced
> 1 tsp curry powder
> 1 tsp salt
> 2 cups dried split green peas, rinsed
> 6 cups vegetable stock
> 2 Tbsp fresh-squeezed lemon juice

Heat the oil in a large stock pot. Sauté the carrot, kale, and onion until tender. Stir in the garlic, curry powder, and salt, and cook 1 minute. Add the rinsed peas and stock and bring to a boil. Reduce the heat, cover, and simmer for 30–40 minutes.

Transfer the pea mixture and the sautéed veggies into a blender (in batches if needed; blender should not be more than half full) and blend to desired consistency.

Add the lemon juice, season with salt and pepper to taste, and serve with a drizzle of olive oil.

Note: Be careful not to fill the blender more than halfway when blending to allow the heated soup room to expand and not overflow.

Tuscan White Bean Quinoa Soup

by Pharmacy In Your Kitchen

Serves 6

This soup is quick to come together, but tastes like it has been simmering all day! It has two of my favorite nutritional power foods, kale and the ancient grain quinoa, both of which are great for brain and overall health. Made easy with the use of a quality basil pesto from the store and canned beans, all you have to do is add the veggies and quinoa and let it simmer.

2 Tbsp olive oil

2 large carrots, peeled and diced

1 small onion, diced

½ cup uncooked quinoa, rinsed and drained

6 cups chicken stock

salt and pepper

¼ cup basil pesto

¼ tsp red pepper flakes

4 whole fresh sage leaves

1 piece of Parmesan rind (optional; remove before serving)

2 cups lacinato (Tuscan) kale, chopped

2 14-oz cans cannellini beans, drained

1 Tbsp lemon zest

3 Tbsp lemon juice

grated Parmesan cheese for serving (optional)

In a soup pot, heat the olive oil over medium heat. Add the carrot and sauté until almost tender, then add the onion. Season with salt and pepper, and sauté until onion is translucent. Add the rinsed and drained quinoa and cook with the carrot and onion mixture until it is slightly toasted and fragrant. Add the stock, pesto, red pepper flakes, sage, kale, beans, and Parmesan rind. Bring to a boil, then reduce to simmer for 30 minutes. Add the lemon zest and juice, and season to taste with salt and pepper. Remove the Parmesan rind before serving. Top with grated Parmesan cheese, if desired.

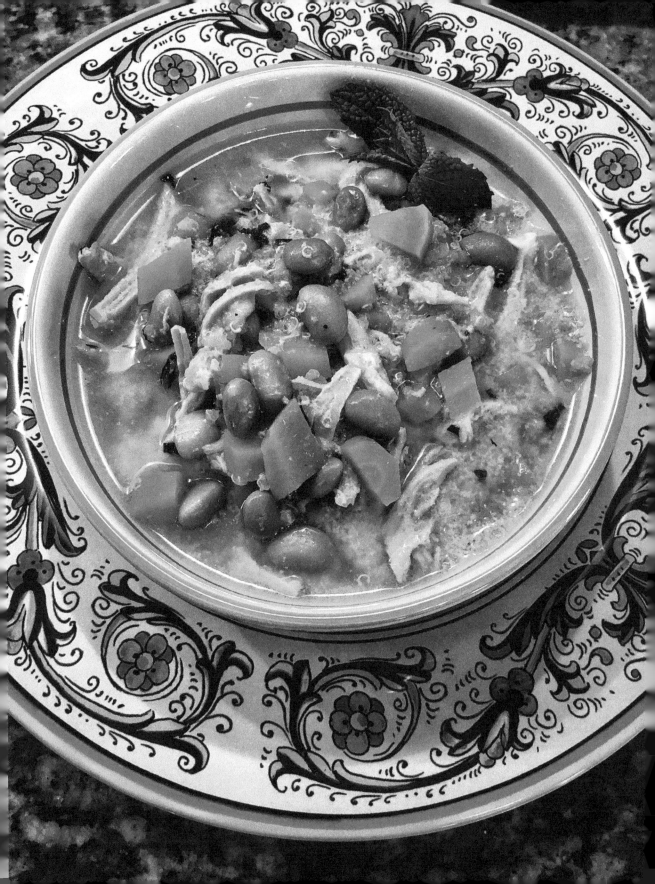

Quinoa Chicken Soup

by Pharmacy In Your Kitchen

Serves 3–4

Several years ago, I had the opportunity to take a cooking class in Peru. Although everything we made in that class was delicious, this recipe has been requested by my family over and over again. It is easy, comforting, and a great use of leftover quinoa (a grain that meets my nutritional standards). I don't typically use a lot of animal protein, but when I do, I buy the best quality I can and use a minimal amount. The small amount of chicken in this recipe is supplemented with edamame, or fava beans, which are anti-inflammatory, high in fiber, and a delicious plant protein.

    1 Tbsp olive oil
    1 cup chopped carrot
    1 cup frozen shelled edamame or fava beans
    ½ tsp minced garlic
    3 cups chicken stock
    1 cup cooked quinoa
    1 cup shredded cooked organic chicken
    2 Tbsp evaporated milk or half-and-half
    1 Tbsp fresh mozzarella cheese, shredded
    ½ tsp chopped cilantro or mint
    salt and pepper
    1 egg

In a soup pot, warm the olive oil over medium heat. Add the carrot, beans, and garlic and sauté several minutes until the carrots are soft. Add the stock and all the other ingredients except the egg. Cover and bring to almost a boil. Once the soup is almost boiling, reduce the heat to a simmer.

In a small bowl, scramble the egg with a fork. Slowly whisk in 1 cup of warm (but not boiling) broth to the egg. Add this egg mixture back to the soup pot while stirring constantly. Season with salt and pepper.

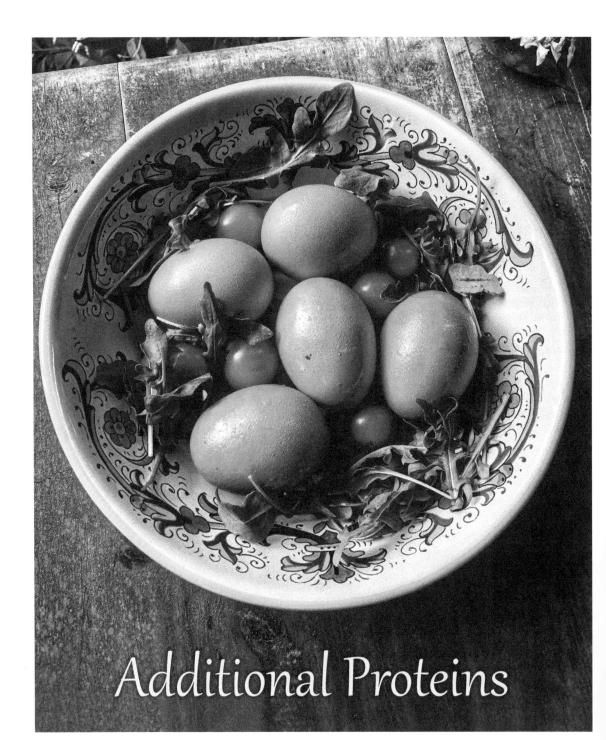

Additional Proteins

Rainbow Roasted Eggs

by Pharmacy In Your Kitchen

Serves 6

I made this for my friends before I had an official name for it. They all loved it and named it for me. I think the name fits. You can easily change the veggies and beans to what you have in your pantry, but this is what I had at the time and it was delicious. I use eggs as naturally sourced as possible and I don't eat them every day, but they do offer B vitamins, which are good for cognitive brain function and mental focus. Combining them with a rainbow of vegetables and cancer-fighting Asian mushrooms makes this a big winner for brain and overall health.

1 large sweet potato, unpeeled (more nutritious that way), diced

1 large white baking potato, unpeeled and diced

4 cups beets, unpeeled and diced

1 cup frozen corn

2 cups cooked black beans or lentils

1 cup shiitake or other Asian mushrooms, chopped

3 Tbsp olive oil

3 cloves garlic, minced

1 tsp chili powder

½ tsp ground cumin

½ tsp smoked paprika

salt and pepper

6 eggs

2 Tbsp cilantro or Italian parsley, chopped

continued . . .

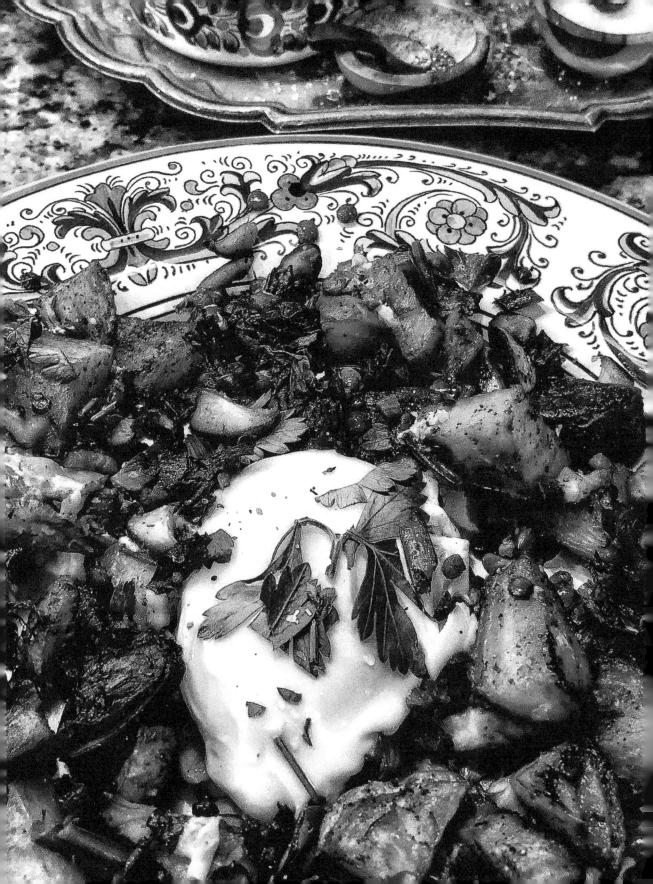

Rainbow Roasted Eggs, continued . . .

In a large plastic bag or bowl, combine the olive oil and all the spices followed by all the veggies and beans. Gently toss to combine and coat well. Arrange on a large baking sheet and roast in 450° oven for 18–22 minutes, depending on the size of your vegetables, stirring halfway through to be sure everything is cooking evenly. Remove from the oven and create 6 pockets for the eggs to be cracked into. Once the eggs are in place, season with salt and pepper and return to the oven for 5–7 minutes, depending on how you like your eggs cooked. Garnish with chopped cilantro or parsley.

Note: This can be prepared ahead to the point where the veggies are roasted, but wait to add the eggs until you are ready to serve. Warm the veggies back up in the oven before adding the eggs.

Halibut over Tarragon Lentils and Sweet Potatoes

by Pharmacy In Your Kitchen

Serves 4

The lentils and sweet potatoes make a delicious side by themselves, packed with plant protein, beta-carotene, and iron. The halibut gives the added benefits of vitamins A and D, and omega-3 fatty acids. All good for your brain, your heart, and your overall health!

1 Tbsp olive oil

1 onion, diced

2 cloves garlic, minced

1 sweet potato, diced*

2½ cups chicken or vegetable broth

1¼ cups green lentils, rinsed

salt and pepper

1 Tbsp olive oil

4 6-oz halibut fillets

¼ cup Dijon mustard

¼ cup dry white wine

¼ cup chicken or vegetable broth

1 Tbsp chopped fresh tarragon

*Sweet potatoes come in three colors: orange, purple, and white. Each color is slightly different in taste and nutrition, so try all three separately, or at the same time for variety and interest.

In a large saucepan, heat 1 Tbsp olive oil over medium heat. Add the onion and cook until softened, about 5 minutes. Add the garlic and sweet potato and cook for an additional minute. Add the broth and lentils, then cover and simmer until the lentils are tender but not overcooked, about 20 minutes. Season with salt and pepper.

In a large skillet, heat the additional 1Tbsp of olive oil over medium heat. Season the fish with salt and pepper and cook until opaque throughout, 3–5 minutes per side.

In a small saucepan, mix together the mustard, wine, and broth. Bring to a boil for about a minute to cook off some of the wine flavor. Remove from heat and stir in the tarragon. Serve the fish on a bed of the lentil/sweet potato mixture and drizzle with the sauce.

Maple Glazed Salmon

by Pharmacy In Your Kitchen

Serves 4

This recipe is great on the grill, but also can be prepared in the oven with the same results. I love the combination of these spices, which provide the benefits of anti-inflammation and better cognitive function, while deliciously flavoring this omega-3-fatty-acid-rich salmon. The touch of maple syrup is a natural way to add a bit of sweetness to complement and round out this wonderful spicy dish.

    2 Tbsp olive oil
    1 Tbsp maple syrup
    2 tsp paprika
    2 tsp chili powder
    1 tsp salt
    ½ tsp cumin
    4 6-oz salmon fillets

Prepare the grill (or if roasting in the oven, heat oven to 450° and line a baking sheet with parchment paper). Combine all ingredients except salmon, and rub mixture on top of the salmon to cover. Grill over medium heat for 7 minutes or until the fish is done to your likeness. If you are roasting in the oven, test with a fork after 10 minutes and continue cooking to your preference. Be careful not to overcook.

Note: Himalayan or other salts that are not refined provide the added benefits of trace minerals.

Shrimp and Grits Reboot with Four Veggies

by Pharmacy In Your Kitchen

Serves 4

I promise you won't even miss the tasso gravy or bacon when you substitute creamy avocado, sautéed spinach, Brussels sprouts, and cherry tomatoes in this southern favorite! It practically melts in your mouth as it nourishes your body with the colors of the rainbow, while still satisfying your desire for shrimp and grits. The addition of all the veggies in this dish changes the nutritional value of a family favorite into a heart-healthy, brain-boosting dish that everyone will enjoy.

4 cups water
1 cup grits
¼ cup milk of choice
1 lb peeled and deveined shrimp
3 Tbsp olive oil, divided
garlic salt
pepper
3 cups shredded Brussels sprouts
6–8 oz fresh baby spinach, chopped
salt and pepper
2 green onions, thinly sliced
1 avocado, cubed
½ cup cherry tomatoes, cut in quarters

Add 1 tsp salt to water and bring to a boil. Add grits, and cook according to package directions. If grits end up too thick, add enough milk to thin them out and add some creaminess.

continued . . .

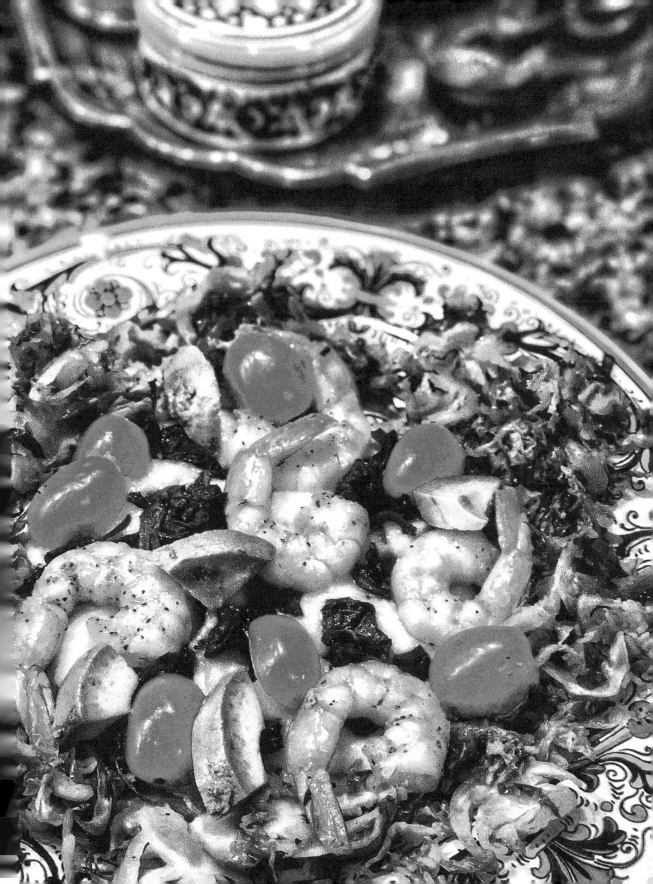

In a large sauté pan over medium heat, sauté the shrimp in 1 Tbsp olive oil and season with garlic salt and pepper. Remove from pan and set aside.

Add 1 Tbsp olive oil and Brussels sprouts to the pan, season with salt and pepper, and sauté until tender, about 6–8 minutes. Remove from pan and set aside.

Add 1 Tbsp olive oil and spinach to the pan and sauté until wilted and tender. Season with salt and pepper.

Place grits on a plate and top with shrimp, Brussels sprouts, and spinach. Garnish with green onions, avocado, and tomatoes.

Shrimp Scampi

by Pharmacy In Your Kitchen

Serves 4

This recipe is an Americanized version of an Italian dish that was one of my father's favorites. It uses shrimp instead of prawns, and adds the nutritional power of garlic and lemon. This makes a wonderful appetizer, but I usually serve it over an ancient grain pasta or forbidden rice. If there are any leftovers (highly doubtful), the flavor is even better the next day.

 1 Tbsp olive oil
 1½ lbs shrimp, peeled and deveined
 3 cloves garlic, minced
 ⅓ cup dry white wine
 ½ tsp salt
 ¼ tsp black pepper
 ¼ cup chopped fresh Italian parsley
 1 Tbsp lemon juice

In a large skillet, warm the olive oil over medium heat. Add the shrimp and sauté 1 minute. Add the garlic, wine, salt, and pepper and bring to a boil. Reduce heat to medium, add the parsley and lemon juice, and toss to combine.

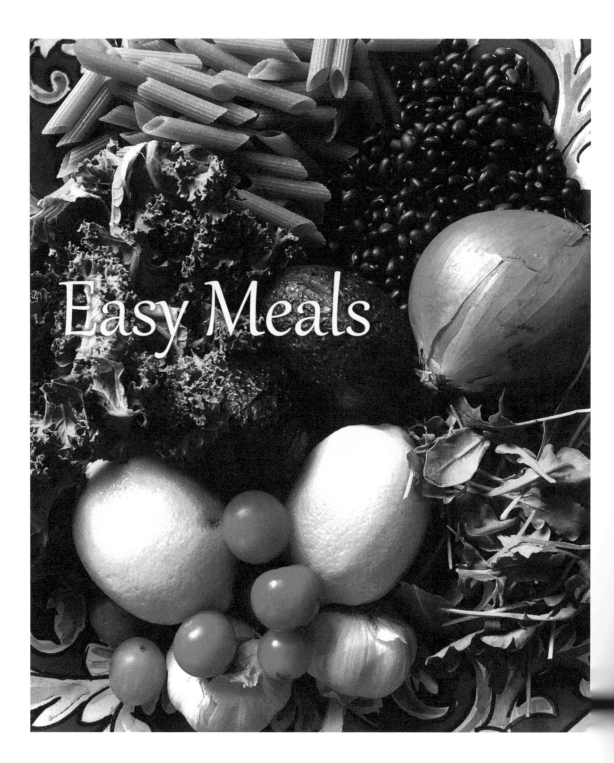

Easy Meals

Rainbow Quinoa "Fried Rice"

adapted from *The Roasted Root*

Serves 4

This is a wonderful recipe to introduce someone to quinoa. Because the grain is high in protein, you can decrease the amount of animal protein in this recipe as I did, or omit it altogether if you choose. Avocado oil has similar health benefits to olive oil, but has a higher flash point so can be used at a higher heat, as in this recipe.

1 cup uncooked quinoa

1 Tbsp avocado oil

2 carrots, peeled and chopped

1 large broccoli crown, chopped

1 zucchini, chopped

2 cups shredded kale

2 tsp fresh ginger, peeled and grated

3 cloves garlic, minced

3 Tbsp soy sauce

1 Tbsp avocado oil

1 cup shredded cooked chicken (optional)

salt and pepper

3 eggs, beaten

sliced green onion to garnish

1 Tbsp toasted sesame seeds (optional)

Rinse the quinoa and cook according to directions in a medium saucepan. Heat oil in a wok or large sauté pan over medium heat. Add all the vegetables and cook to desired tenderness. Stir in the ginger and garlic and cook another minute or so. Add the cooked quinoa, soy sauce, remaining avocado oil, chicken, and salt and pepper, and stir gently to combine. In a smaller pan, scramble the eggs as desired and cut into strips. Add to the quinoa and garnish with green onion and sesame seeds.

Butternut Squash Porter Chili

adapted from *Oh My Veggies*

Serves 6

I love this seasonal fall recipe. It is hearty as you would expect chili to be, and it provides the nutritional benefits of the winter squash and black beans, allowing you to decrease your animal protein and not even miss it. Most of the antioxidant flavonoids are often found in the outer layers of onions, so try not to overpeel them before you dice them. This dish is delicious served over rice or pasta. I suggest using ancient grain pasta for the added benefits of the ancient grains over traditional wheat.

1 Tbsp olive oil

1 medium onion, diced

1 butternut squash, peeled, seeded, and cubed (about 4 cups)*

2 Tbsp chili powder

1 Tbsp ground cumin

½ tsp ground coriander**

12 oz porter beer

1 28-oz can diced tomatoes

2 15-oz cans black beans, rinsed and drained

½ tsp salt

¼ tsp pepper

chopped avocado

chopped green onions

hot sauce

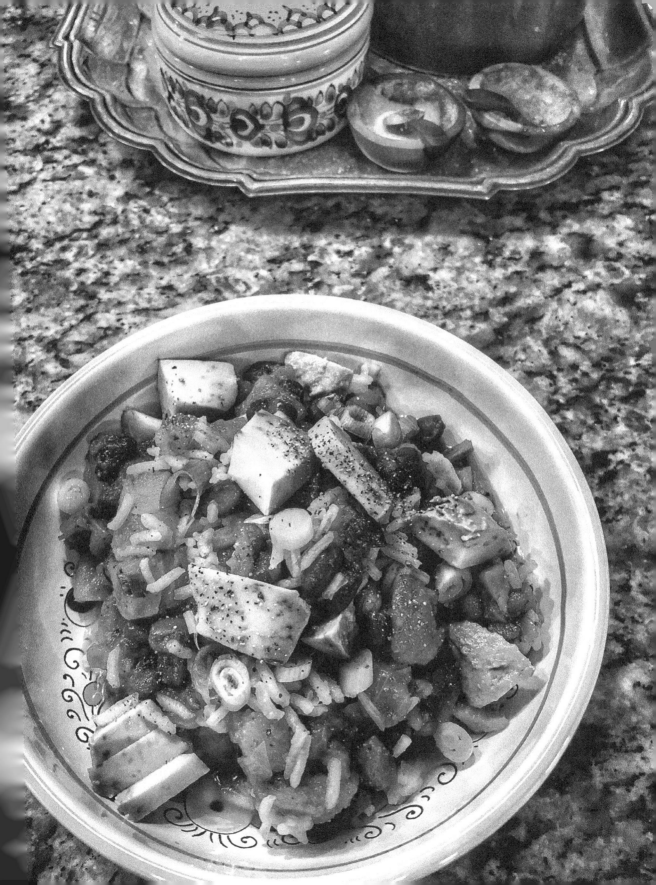

Butternut Squash Porter Chili, continued . . .

In a soup pot, warm the oil, and sauté the onion until translucent. Add the squash and the spices and cook a few more minutes, stirring until well combined. Add the remaining ingredients and bring to a simmer. Cover and continue to cook for at least 1 hour (the longer it simmers, the better the flavor).

Serve over rice or grain of choice, and garnish as desired with diced avocado, chopped green onions, and a dash of hot sauce.

*To save time, look for precut butternut squash.

**If you do not enjoy the taste of coriander, you can substitute caraway seeds. When I do this, I add 2 tsp maple syrup to help bring the natural sweetness together in this dish.

Sugar Snap Pea and Asparagus Pasta

by Pharmacy In Your Kitchen

Serves 4

This is an example of how you can bump up the nutritional value of something you love, i.e., pasta, with a few delicious swaps. Use either an ancient grain pasta or bean pasta, and replace the meat sauce with two green veggies that offer plant protein, fiber, and vitamins. The fresh tomatoes and a small amount of good-quality cheese bring everything together for a pasta dish you can feel good about eating that nourishes your body and brain.

    1 lb asparagus, trimmed and cut into 1-inch pieces

    ½ lb ancient grain or bean-based pasta*

    ½ lb sugar snap peas, trimmed

    ¼ cup Italian dressing or vinaigrette of choice

    1 cup halved cherry tomatoes

    ½ cup freshly grated Parmesan cheese

    salt and pepper

Bring a large pot of salted water to a boil. Add the asparagus and cook until crisp-tender. (This will only take a few minutes and depends on the thickness of the asparagus.) Remove asparagus from the boiling water using a slotted spoon and place in a bowl of cool water. Cool the asparagus slightly and drain. Bring the water in the pot back to a boil. Add the pasta and cook 2 minutes less than the package directions, then add in the sugar snap peas and boil for remaining 2 minutes. Add the asparagus back in the pot just to warm up. Reserve about a cup of pasta water for possible use later to loosen the pasta up a bit. Drain the pasta and veggies well and return to the pot. Add the dressing, and salt and pepper to taste. (If the pasta needs more liquid, add a small amount of pasta cooking water a little at a time, or additional dressing to taste.) Lightly toss in the tomatoes and sprinkle with cheese.

*Instead of white flour-based pasta, I use a higher protein higher fiber ancient grain or bean pasta like chickpea (garbanzo bean), or lentils. There are many choices out there, so experiment and find some you like.

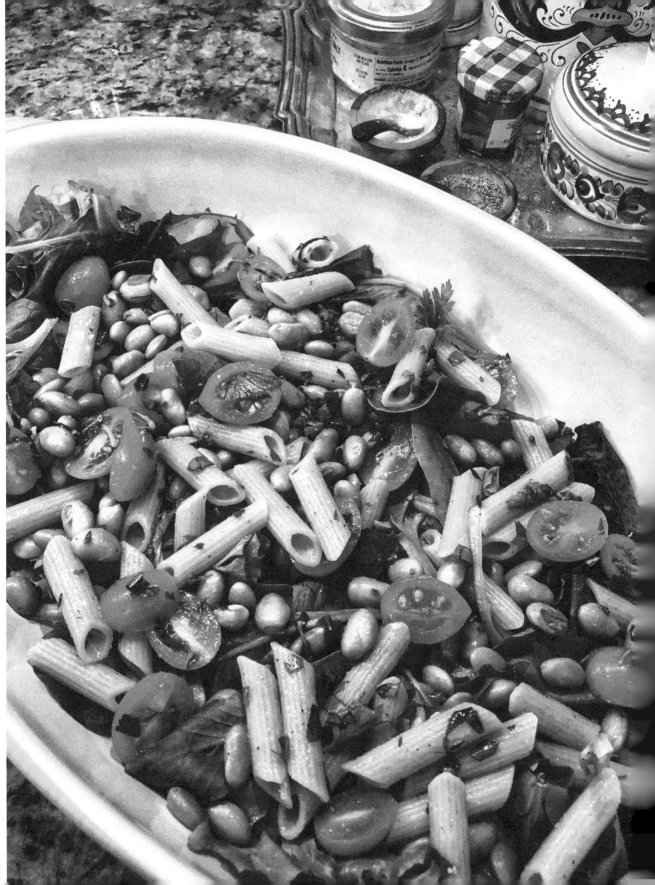

Pasta Salad with Edamame, Arugula, and Herbs

adapted from *Cooking Light*

Serves 4

This pasta salad is actually more of a "salad with pasta," which is exactly why it is rich in nutrients and beautiful colors—perfect for eating the rainbow. The darker the color, the richer the nutrients, so the bright green of the edamame, combined with the arugula, parsley, thyme, and basil, and the bright red tomatoes come together to offer a plant-based protein salad that is heart healthy and brain boosting. It also happens to be delicious.

    8 oz uncooked ancient grain or bean pasta*
    3 Tbsp olive oil
    2 cups frozen shelled edamame, thawed
    2 cups loosely packed arugula (or mixed greens)
    1 cup halved grape tomatoes
    ¼ cup chopped fresh Italian parsley
    ¼ cup fresh-squeezed lemon juice
    3 Tbsp chopped fresh basil
    1 Tbsp chopped fresh thyme
    salt and pepper
    2 oz freshly grated Parmesan cheese (optional)

Cook pasta according to package directions, then drain. In a large skillet, heat oil over medium heat. Add edamame and cook until thoroughly heated, about 2 minutes. In a large bowl combine pasta and edamame. Stir in the arugula, tomatoes, lemon juice and all the herbs. Season with salt and pepper to taste. If desired, sprinkle with a small amount of cheese before serving.

*Instead of white flour-based pasta, I use a higher-protein, higher-fiber ancient grain or bean (chickpea or lentil) pasta. There are many choices out there, so experiment and find some you like.

Salad Pizza

by Pharmacy In Your Kitchen

Serves 2

This is a perfect example of how you can transform a recipe for a favorite food into something similar but nutritiously better. We all love pizza, but this one is made with a rainbow of vegetables, hummus, and shrimp. The shrimp is rich in B vitamins, which help with cognitive functioning, the chickpeas are full of antioxidants, and the more veggies you can pack on the better! When I can find it, I use sprouted or naturally fermented breads and grains. They are easier for your body to digest, and therefore the nutrients are more bioavailable. Do the best you can with the choices you have. You'll note there are no ingredient amounts listed for this recipe; just use as much of each as looks good to you!

   Flatbread of choice (such as Lavash Roll Up, sprouted and naturally fermented)
   Hummus of choice
   Mixed salad made with as many different colors of the rainbow as possible
   Dressing of choice
   Cooked shrimp, chopped
   Cherry tomatoes, quartered

Cut flatbread into manageable pieces and toast at 450° for 4 minutes.

Spread toasted flatbread with a thick layer of hummus. Top with lightly dressed rainbow salad. Top with shrimp and cherry tomatoes.

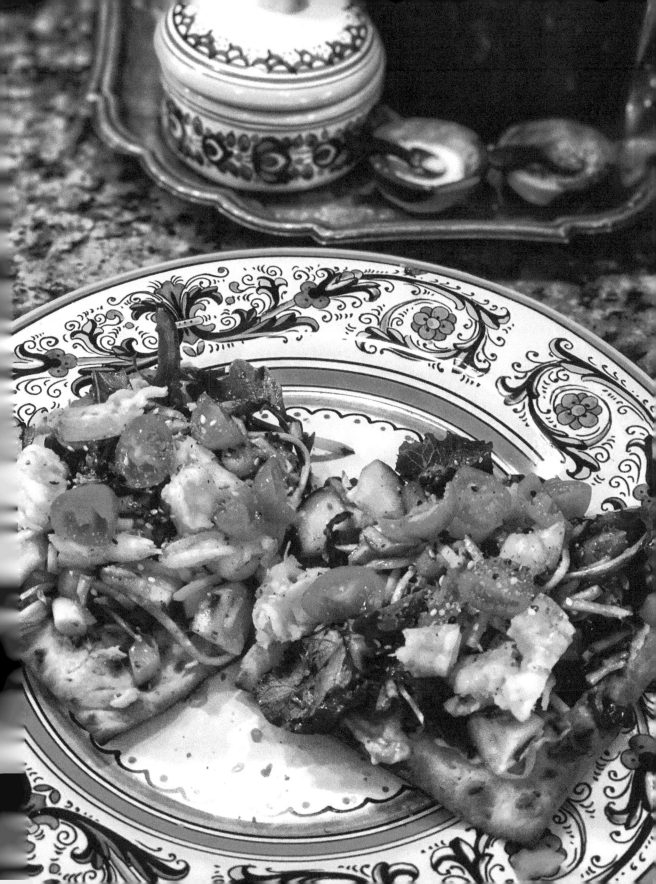

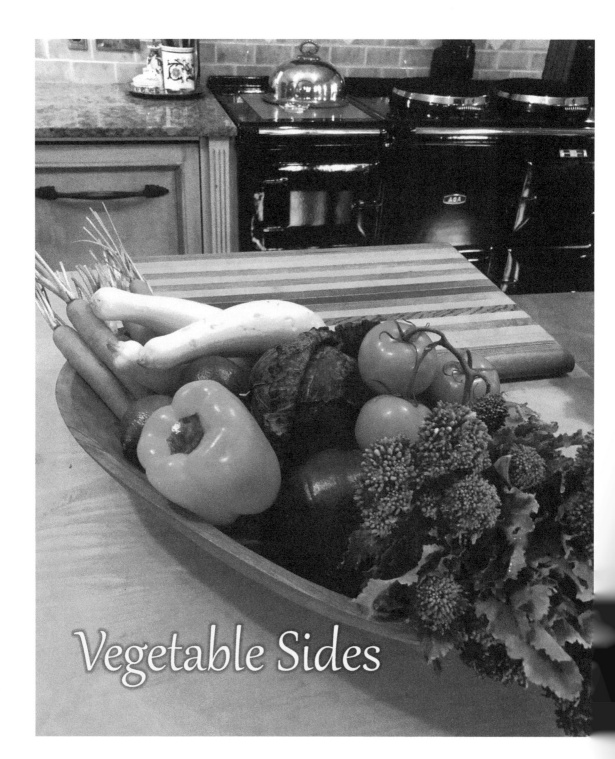

Vegetable Sides

Avocado Strawberry Tomato Salad

by Pharmacy In Your Kitchen

Serves 3–4

This is a beautiful salad that reminds me to eat seasonally and take advantage of all the nutrients that grow in the spring and into the summer. Eating seasonally means that you will be getting a variety of fruits and vegetables in your diet, and that is the best way to ensure you are getting what your body needs throughout the year. This recipe comes together very quickly and is a delicious way to help your mental focus and overall health.

> 1 cup sliced strawberries
> 1 cup halved cherry tomatoes
> 1 avocado, pitted and diced
> ⅓ cup pecans, toasted
> ⅓ cup loosely packed basil, torn
> olive oil
> salt and pepper
> balsamic glaze*

Place the strawberries, tomatoes, avocado, and basil in a shallow bowl. Drizzle with olive oil, and season with salt and pepper. Gently toss. Drizzle with balsamic glaze.

*Balsamic glaze is reduced and thickened balsamic vinegar and is readily available at most grocery stores.

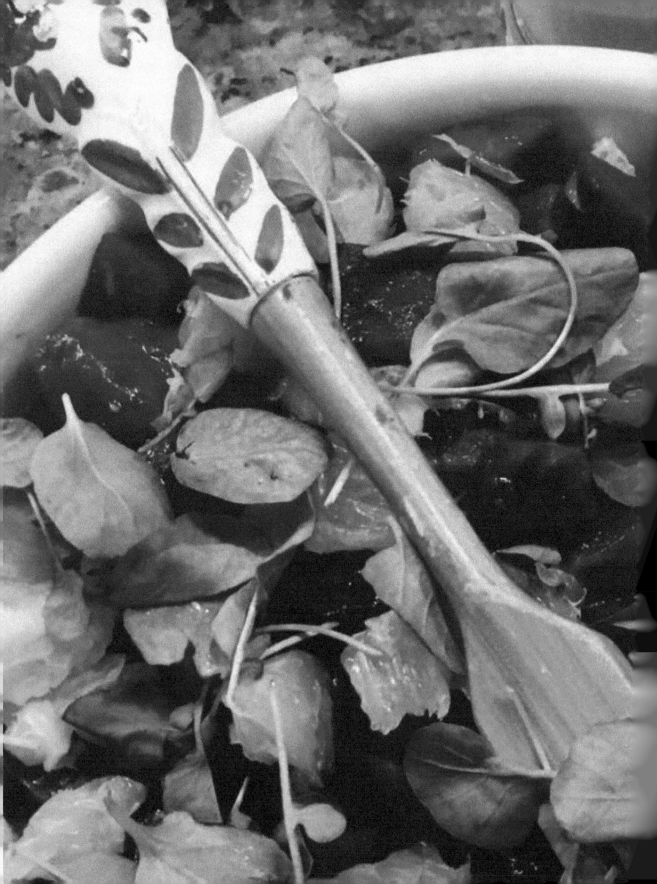

Roasted Beets with Citrus and Greens

by Pharmacy In Your Kitchen

Serves 4

I made this delicious recipe for Thanksgiving a few years ago, wanting to change our traditional plates a bit, and bring more color and variety of nutrients to the table. It was a big hit, and everyone welcomed the change and new flavors of this dish. The beets are full of fiber and nitrites, and balance nicely with the vitamin C-rich oranges and the nutrient-rich dark greens. Topping everything off with toasted walnuts or pistachios makes this a delicious addition to any winter meal.

    6 medium beets, unpeeled
    olive oil
    2 navel oranges, divided
    balsamic vinegar
    juice of half a lemon
    handful of watercress, arugula, or micro greens
    salt and pepper
    ¼ cup toasted and chopped walnuts or pistachios

Wash beets and remove the tops and bottoms. Cut beets into bite-sized cubes. Place beets on a baking sheet lined with parchment paper and toss with olive oil, salt, and pepper. Roast at 450° for 25–30 minutes or until tender. Remove from oven, place beets in a large bowl, and let cool.

Zest one orange and set zest aside. In a separate small bowl, peel and carefully section the orange to remove each membrane and discard any pith.

Drizzle some olive oil and balsamic vinegar over the cooled beets. Add the lemon juice and the juice of half an orange. Season with salt and pepper and the reserved orange zest. Chill until ready to serve, then toss in the orange segments, greens, and nuts.

Kale and Brussels Sprout Caesar Salad

adapted from *Just a Taste*

Serves 4

This is a nutrient-packed version of a traditional Caesar salad. By substituting kale and Brussels sprouts for the lettuce, you get the added nutritional benefit of two powerhouses for the body. Add in the walnuts, wonderful for the heart and brain, and nutritional yeast, which is full of B vitamins and good for overall health, and you have a winningly delicious combination. This salad also holds up well once dressed in the unlikely case that you have any leftovers.

Dressing:
2 Tbsp Dijon mustard
1 Tbsp minced shallots
1½ tsp lemon zest
¼ cup fresh-squeezed lemon juice
2 tsp honey
1 clove garlic, minced
¼ cup olive oil
salt and pepper
4 cups shredded lacinato (Tuscan) kale
4 cups finely shredded Brussels sprouts
½ cup chopped toasted walnuts
1–2 Tbsp nutritional yeast

In a small bowl, combine the mustard, shallots, lemon juice and zest, honey, and garlic. Then whisk in the olive oil to make a smooth dressing. Season to taste with salt and pepper.

In a large bowl, combine the remaining ingredients and toss with as much dressing as you like. (The remainder can be used for additional salads or as a marinade.)

Helpful Hint: Always zest your lemons before squeezing them for juice. This allows you to use the same lemon for both purposes.

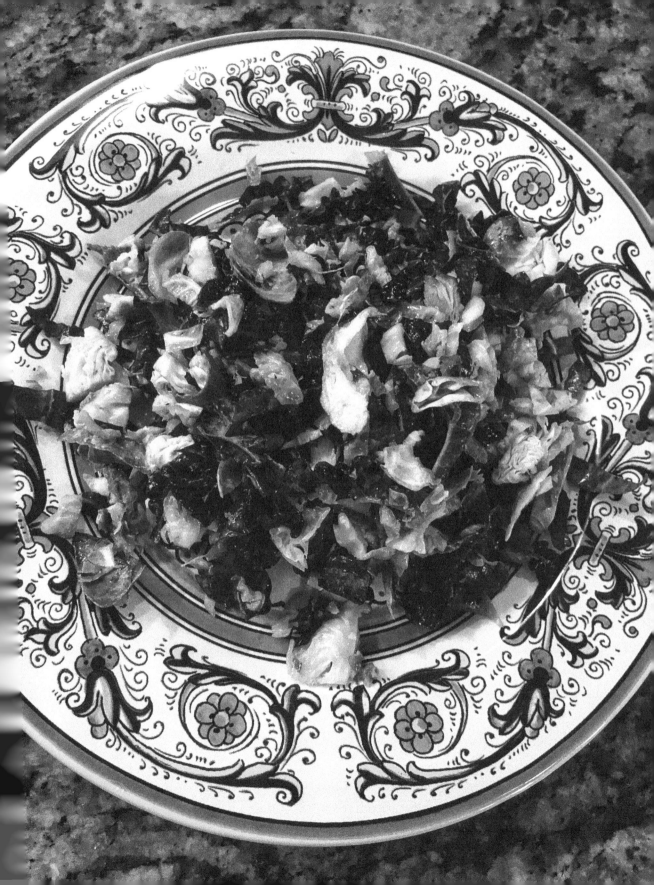

Ginger Miso Slaw

adapted from *Love and Lemons*

Serves 4

This beautiful and colorful slaw is packed with the nutrients of summer herbs and peaches. It also has cabbage (a cruciferous powerhouse), miso (fermented soybeans), and memory-boosting ginger. It is a good example of how easy it is to incorporate something fermented into your diet, something we should be doing on a regular basis to keep our guts healthy!

Dressing:
¼ cup almond butter
2 Tbsp white miso paste
2 Tbsp lime juice
1 tsp toasted sesame oil
1 tsp fresh grated ginger
½–1 tsp sriracha or other hot sauce
4 Tbsp water
7 cups shredded cabbage
2 green onions, chopped
½ cup chopped cilantro
½ cup torn fresh basil
salt and pepper
¼ cup toasted sesame seeds
1 peach, thinly sliced

In a small bowl, mix the almond butter, miso paste, lime juice, sesame oil, and ginger, and season to taste with sriracha or hot sauce. Whisk in the water.

In a large bowl, combine the cabbage, green onions, cilantro, and basil, and toss with the dressing. Add the sliced peaches and sesame seeds and season to taste with salt and pepper.

Roasted Butternut Squash with Tahini Dressing and Pomegranate

by Pharmacy In Your Kitchen

Serves 4

This beautiful winter dish comes together quickly and provides so many nutrients that your body needs to be healthy and strong. The beta-carotene from the butternut squash, iron in the roasted sesame seeds in the tahini, B vitamins from superfood pomegranate, and vitamins C, K, and A from the arugula are just some of the reasons why this dish is a seasonal winner. All these powerful ingredients combine to make a delicious and nutritious dish that will not disappoint, and will nourish your body as well.

24 oz peeled and diced fresh butternut squash
2 Tbsp olive oil
¼ tsp salt
¼ tsp pepper
1 cup arugula or watercress
½ cup pomegranate seeds

Dressing:
4 tsp tahini paste
1 Tbsp fresh-squeezed lemon juice
1 Tbsp olive oil
1 Tbsp water

Line a large rimmed baking sheet with parchment paper. Place butternut squash on the sheet and toss with the olive oil to coat, season with salt and pepper, and spread evenly in the pan. Roast at 450° for 35–40 minutes or until browned, stirring halfway through.

Combine the tahini paste, lemon juice, remaining olive oil, and water in a small bowl and whisk to make a smooth dressing. In a large bowl gently toss together the cooked squash, arugula, and pomegranate seeds. Drizzle with the tahini dressing.

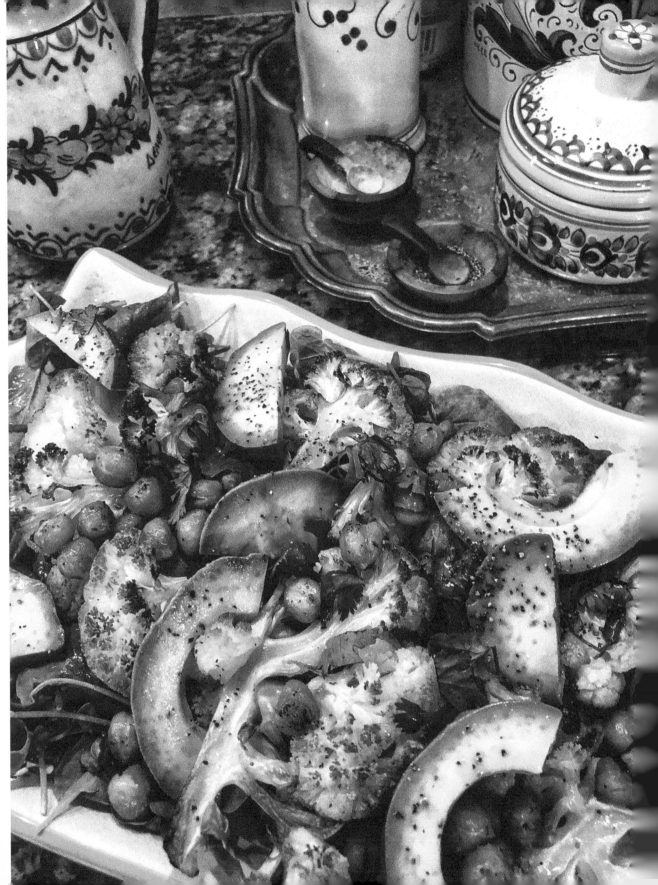

Roasted Cauliflower and Chickpea Salad

by Pharmacy In Your Kitchen

Serves 2–3

There are three impressive characters in this salad. First is cauliflower, a cruciferous vegetable in the cabbage family that has powerful cancer-fighting nutrients, as well as antioxidants and folate, which are wonderful for brain health. The chickpeas are high in protein and rich in folate and magnesium, and delicious roasted in this recipe, adding an unexpected crunch to the salad. Finally, the avocado brings healthy fats to the table, and provides a creaminess like only avocado can.

1 head of cauliflower cut into ½-inch-thick "steaks"
¼ cup olive oil
1 tsp salt
½ tsp cumin
¼ tsp pepper
¼ tsp garlic salt
dash cayenne pepper
1 15-oz can chickpeas, rinsed and drained
1 avocado, sliced
2 Tbsp chopped fresh cilantro
mixed dark greens

Dressing:
¼ cup olive oil
2 Tbsp fresh squeezed lemon juice
1½ Tbsp water
1 tsp tahini
½ tsp maple syrup

continued . . .

Roasted Cauliflower and Chickpea Salad, continued . . .

Wash the cauliflower and remove the bulky part of the stem and outer leaves, but keep the head intact. Slice the head lengthwise into flat "steaks."

In a small bowl, combine the oil, salt, cumin, pepper, garlic salt, and cayenne. Put the cauliflower on a large sheet pan lined with foil or parchment. Drizzle half the olive oil mixture over the cauliflower and toss to mix well. Mix chickpeas in with remaining oil mixture and set aside. Roast cauliflower at 450° for 20 minutes. Remove from oven, turn steaks with a spatula, and add chickpeas to pan. Return to the oven for 20 minutes.

In a small bowl, whisk together olive oil, lemon juice, water, tahini, and maple syrup.

On a large platter make a bed of dark salad greens, and top with roasted cauliflower and chickpeas. Garnish with sliced avocado, chopped cilantro, and drizzle with dressing as desired.

Roasted Root Vegetables with Orange, Ginger, and Turmeric

adapted from *The Roasted Root*

Serves 4

This is one of my absolute favorite roasted vegetable recipes. The flavor combination of the garlic, ginger, turmeric, oregano, rosemary, and thyme is so delicious, and rich in powerful nutrients that are so good for your overall health and brain function. If you can't find black garlic (fermented), just substitute regular. This dish is easy, colorful, anti-inflammatory, and full of antioxidants to keep you healthy and well nourished.

Dressing:
4 cloves mashed black garlic*
¼ cup olive oil
2 Tbsp balsamic vinegar
1 Tbsp maple syrup
1 Tbsp fresh ginger, peeled and grated
2 tsp orange zest
¼ tsp ground turmeric
1 tsp dried oregano
1 tsp dried rosemary
1 tsp dried thyme leaves
1 tsp salt
pepper to taste

1 15-oz can chickpeas, drained
4 beets, washed and chopped in 1-inch pieces, (skin left on)
6 carrots (rainbow colors, preferably), peeled and chopped in 1-inch pieces
1 large sweet potato, chopped in uniform 1-inch pieces,
1 onion, sliced

continued . . .

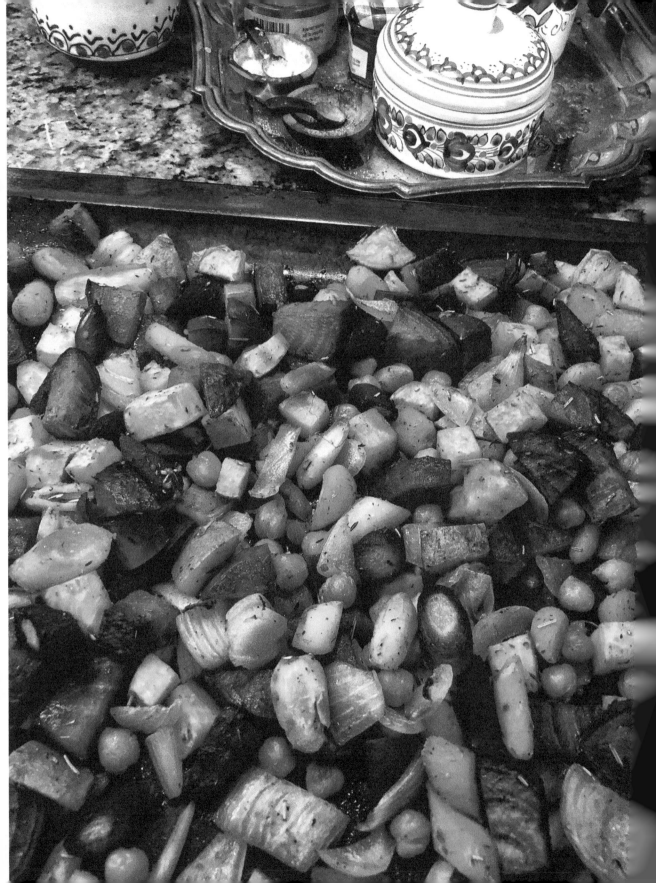

Roasted Root Vegetables with Orange, Ginger, and Turmeric, continued . . .

In a blender, combine the garlic, oil, vinegar, maple syrup, ginger, orange zest, spices, salt, and pepper until smooth. Toss the vegetables and chickpeas with the dressing on a rimmed baking sheet and roast for 30 minutes in a 450° oven, stirring halfway through to be sure everything cooks evenly. Yum!

*Black garlic is fermented, which is good for your gut health, and has a wonderful flavor if you can find it. Otherwise, substitute regular garlic.

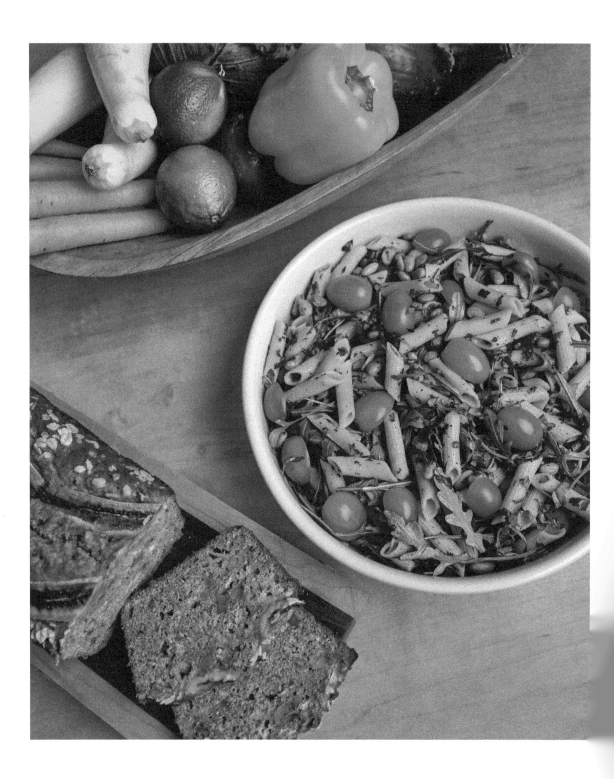

Sample Weekly Eating Plan

Monday

BREAKFAST: Tomato, Kale, and Herb Baked Eggs

SNACK: a piece of seasonal fruit

LUNCH: Kale and Brussels Sprouts Caesar Salad

SNACK: seasonal veggies and hummus

DINNER: Tuscan White Bean Quinoa Soup and a side salad

Tuesday

BREAKFAST: Baked Blueberry Coconut Oatmeal

SNACK: handful of almonds or walnuts

LUNCH: leftover Tuscan White Bean Quinoa Soup

SNACK: Nutritiously Delicious Granola

DINNER: Pasta Salad with Edamame, Arugula, and Herbs and Ginger Miso Slaw

Wednesday

BREAKFAST: Honey Walnut Banana Oat Bread

SNACK: a piece of seasonal fruit

LUNCH: leftover Pasta Salad with Edamame, Arugula, and Herbs

SNACK: leftover Ginger Miso Slaw

DINNER: Butternut Squash Porter Chili

Thursday

BREAKFAST: Overnight Oats with Chia, Carrots, and Raisins

SNACK: a piece of seasonal fruit

LUNCH: leftover Butternut Squash Porter Chili

SNACK: slice of leftover Honey Walnut Banana Oat Bread

DINNER: Kale and Quinoa Super Salad and Roasted Root Vegetables with Orange, Ginger, and Turmeric

Friday

BREAKFAST: Nutritiously Delicious Granola with almond milk

SNACK: piece of seasonal fruit

LUNCH: Power Salad with Ancient Grains and Berries

SNACK: leftover Roasted Root Vegetables with Orange, Ginger, and Turmeric

DINNER: Maple Glazed Salmon with Roasted Cauliflower and Chickpea Salad

Saturday

BREAKFAST: Blueberry Walnut Breakfast Cookies

SNACK: seasonal berries

LUNCH: make a rainbow salad with all the colors of the rainbow and dress with Healthy Vinaigrette

SNACK: leftover Roasted Cauliflower and Chickpea Salad

DINNER: Salad Pizza and Quick as a Wink Spinach Lentil Soup

Sunday

BREAKFAST: Banana Almond Butter Roll-Ups

SNACK: leftover Nutritiously Delicious Granola

LUNCH: leftover Quick as a Wink Spinach Lentil Soup

SNACK: seasonal veggies and hummus

DINNER: Shrimp and Grits Reboot and a side salad

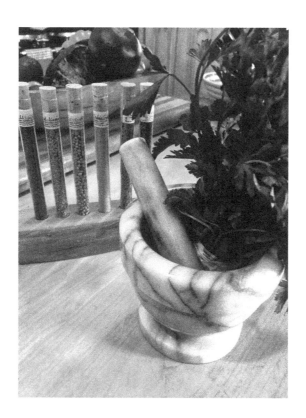

References

1. Graham Simpson, *Well Man: Live Longer by Controlling Inflammation* (Laguna Beach, CA: Basic Health Publication, 2010), 1.
2. Dale E. Bredesen, *The End of Alzheimer's* (New York: Avery, 2017), 5.
3. Bredesen, 10.
4. Gill Livingston et al. "Dementia prevention, intervention, and care," *The Lancet* 390, no. 10113 (July 19, 2017): 2673–2734, https://doi.org/10.1016/S0140-6736(17)31363-6.
5. Barry Reisberg, The Global Deterioration Scale for Assessment of Primary Degenerative Dementia.
6. Ashley Marcin, "What Causes Menopause Brain Fog and How's It Treated?," Healthline, December 22, 2017, https://www.healthline.com/health/menopause/menopause-brain-fog.
7. M. T. Weber, L. H. Rubin, P. M. Maki. "Cognition in perimenopause: the effect of transition stage," *Menopause* 20, no. 5 (May 2013): 511–517, https://www.ncbi.nlm.nih.gov/pubmed/23615642.
8. Quishan Tao et al. "Association of Chronic Low-grade Inflammation with Risk of Alzheimer Disease in ApoE4 Carriers," *JAMA Network Open*, October 19, 2018, https://doi.org/10.1001/jamanetworkopen.2018.3597.
9. Karen Weintraub, "For Alzheimer's Sufferers, Brain Inflammation Ignites a Neuron-Killing Forest Fire," *Scientific American*, March 4, 2019.
10. Steven R. Gundry, *The Longevity Paradox* (New York: Harper Collins Publishers, 2019), 37.
11. Betsy Mills, "Does Obesity Increase Dementia Risk?" *Cognitive Vitality* blog, November 8, 2018, https://www.alzdiscovery.org/cognitive-vitality/blog/does-obesity-increase-dementia-risk.

12. Matthew Walker, *Why We Sleep: Unlocking the Power of Sleep and Dreams* (New York: Scribner, 2017), 1.

13. Anton Sirota et al, "Communication between neocortex and hippocampus during sleep in rodents," *PNAS* 100, no. 4 (February 18, 2003): 2065–2069, https://doi.org/10.1073/pnas.0437938100.

14. Lisa Marshall and Jan Born, "The contribution of sleep to hippocampus-dependent memory consolidation," *Trends in Cognitive Sciences* 11, no. 10 (October 1, 2007): 442–450, https://doi.org/10.1016/j.tics.2007.09.001.

15. Boston University Medical Center, "Link found between concussions, Alzheimer's disease," *Science Daily*, January 12, 2017, https://www.sciencedaily.com/releases/2017/01/170112110804.htm.

16. Annie Sneed, "DDT, other Environmental Toxins Linked to Late-Onset Alzheimer's Disease," *Scientific American*, February 10, 2014, https://www.scientificamerican.com/article/studies-link-ddt-other-environmental-toxins-to-late-onset-alzheimers-disease/.

17. Sneed.

18. Peter H. Diamandis and Steven Kotler, Bold: *How to Go Big, Create Wealth, and Impact the World*, (New York: Simon and Schuster, 2015), ix.

19. W. A. Rocca et al, "Hysterectomy, Oophorectomy, Estrogen, and the Risk of Dementia." *Neurodegenerative Diseases* 10 (2012): 175–178, https://doi.org/10.1159/000334764.

20. Lee W. Jones, "Efficacy and Mechanisms of Exercise as Treatment of Cancer," Annual Meeting of the German, Austrian and Swiss Associations for Hematology and Medical Oncology, Basel, October 9–13, 2015.

21. Tim, Ferriss, *Tools of Titans: The Tactics, Routines, and Habits of Billionaires, Icons, and World-Class Performers* (Boston: Houghton, Mifflin Harcourt, 2017), xx.

Suggested Reading and Further Resources

Healthy Living:

Breseden, Dale E. *The End of Alzheimer's*. New York: Avery, 2017.

Brown, Ronald. *The Youth Effect*. St. Augustine, FL: Fine Books Publishing Compan 2007.

Campbell, T. Colin and Thomas M. Campbell II. *The China Study*. Dallas: BenBell Books, 2016.

Emmons, Henry and David Alter. *Staying Sharp*. New York: Touchstone, 2015.

Ferris, Tim. *Tools of Titans*. New York: Houghton Mifflin Harcourt, 2017.

Fotuhi, Majid. *Boost Your Brain*. New York: Harper One, 2013.

Gundry, Steven R. *The Longevity Paradox*. New York: Harper Collins Publishers, 2019

Jebelli, Joseph. *In Pursuit of Memory*. New York: Little Brown and Company, 2017.

Mukherjee, Siddhartha. *The Gene*. New York: Scribner, 2016.

Small, Gary and Gigi Vorgan. *The Alzheimer's Prevention Program*. New York: Workma Publishing, 2012.

Woollen, T. Hayes. *Fuel Your Body, Feed Your Mind*. Seattle, WA: CreateSpace, 2013

Healthy Eating:

Liddon, Angela. *The Oh She Glows Cookbook*. New York: Penguin Group, 2014.

Donofrio, Jeanine and Jack Matthews. *Love and Lemons Every Day*. New York: Penguin Random House, 2019.

Hyman, Mark. *Food Fix*. New York: Little Brown Spark, 2020.

Li, William W. *Eat to Beat Disease*. New York: Grand Central, 2019.

Lipman, Frank and Danielle Claro. *The New Health Rules*. New York: Artisan, 2014.

Lipsky, Sally. *Beyond Cancer*. Charleston, SC: Wellness Ink Publishing, 2018.

McDonald, Patricia. *The ApoE Gene Diet*. Danville, CA: T Penscott Medical Corporation, 2007.

Websites:

bluezones.com

forksoverknives.com

loveandlemons.com

monkeyandmekitchenadventures.com

plantstrong.com

Acknowledgments

*M*any people were involved in the writing of *Healthy Living for a Sharper Mind*. Our sincere appreciation is extended to the many patients, clients, friends, and families we have had the opportunity to work with over the years. They are the inspiration for this book.

Special thanks to Betsy Thorpe for her guidance and encouragement, and for keeping us on task. Thank you to our copyeditor, Maya Myers; our book designer, Diana Wade; and our cover photographer, Rusty Williams. We want to give special recognition to the physicians and staff of Memory and Movement Charlotte who work tirelessly every day with patients and families who are dealing with Alzheimer's disease and Parkinson's. Dr. Chuck Edwards is our hero and a true friend. He continues to teach us the meaning of compassion and empathy and is one of the most caring doctors we know. Thanks to Dr. KD Weeks for his lifelong mentoring and friendship. And to Dr. Chasse Bailey-Dorton, thank you for inspiring and encouraging Pharmacy In Your Kitchen from the very beginning. We want to thank Hayden Hilke, DPT, who lives with her family in Jackson Hole, Wyoming, and started Watershed Jackson, a nonprofit organization that benefits athletes with traumatic brain and spinal-cord injuries. And thanks to Carter and Mark for their literary and artistic guidance. Thank you to Hunter for your inspiring words and helpful edits. And thank you to Susan for always being there.

Lastly, we want to thank our parents, Tom and Velva and Ann and Dave, for always being there and for providing a lifetime of love and encouragement.

About the Authors

Hayes Woollen, MD, MBA

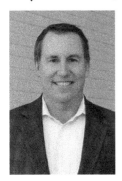
Dr. Hayes Woollen is a primary care physician and experienced healthcare leader with a passion for advanced wellness and neuro-cognitive health. He lives in Charlotte, North Carolina, with his wife, Susan, their three children, and their two Labradors. He is a graduate of Davidson College, received his medical degree from Wake Forest University, and received his MBA at the University of Massachusetts, Amherst.

Cheryl Hoover, RPh

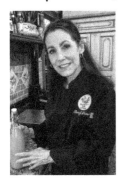
Cheryl Hoover is a registered pharmacist, who after a cancer diagnosis became certified in plant-based nutrition. She believes that there is a Pharmacy In Your Kitchen that you should use every day to prevent disease and be healthy. This book shares the Pharmacy In Your Kitchen philosophy and forty recipes that follow her principles.

If you would like more encouragement on your wellness path, her website is pharmacyinyourkitchen.com. You can also find her on Instagram @pharmacy.in.your.kitchen and Facebook @pharmacyinyourkitchen.

CPSIA information can be obtained
at www.ICGtesting.com
Printed in the USA
LVHW070739210221
679525LV00003B/57

9 780999 430